D1526273

DEMENTIA

DEMENTIA

A survey of the syndrome
of dementia

by

B. Mahendra

Institute of Psychiatry, London
and
Northwick Park Hospital
Harrow, Middlesex

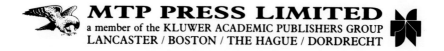

MTP PRESS LIMITED
a member of the KLUWER ACADEMIC PUBLISHERS GROUP
LANCASTER / BOSTON / THE HAGUE / DORDRECHT

Published in the UK and Europe by
MTP Press Limited
Falcon House
Lancaster, England

British Library Cataloguing in Publication Data

Mahendra, B.
  Dementia.
  1. Dementia
  I. Title
  616.89   RC524

  ISBN 0–85200–863–5

Published in the USA by
MTP Press
A division of Kluwer Boston Inc
190 Old Derby Street
Hingham, MA 02043, USA

Library of Congress Cataloguing in Publication Data

Mahendra, B. (Bala), 1950–
  Dementia : a survey of the syndrome of dementia.

  Bibliography: p.
  Includes index.
  1. Dementia.   I. Title.   [DNLM: 1. Dementia.
WM 220 M214d]
  RC521.M34 1984   616.89'82'009   84–14333
  ISBN 0–85200–863–5

Phototypesetting by David John Services Ltd,
Maidenhead, Berks.

Printed in Great Britain by Cradley Print plc, Warley, West Midlands.

Contents

Preface

Three points must strike anyone who has embarked on a study of dementia over a period of time. *Firstly,* that our conception of the syndrome is in a state of flux. Gone, for instance, in the past decade or two, is the requirement of a chronic, progressive, irreversible disorder for the diagnosis. I remember the surgeon who, when I was a student, returned a referral saying he would operate on the man when his dementia got better. Feeling superior, and encouraged by the consultant psychiatrist, we students laughed a good deal at this. Before we finished clerking on that Unit a visiting Professor of Psychiatry had demonstrated the reversibility of the symptoms of dementia in a patient with a rare metabolic disorder. Perhaps ignorance is sometimes an advance on received wisdom. The lesson is the concept of dementia must always reflect the state of knowledge and is therefore in a sense *ad hoc.*

Secondly, what the criteria for, and also who the arbiters of, the diagnosis might be is not always clear. It is traditional to think that expressing opinions and making diagnosis of mental illness is almost a civic right, i.e. virtually everyone's business. It would be an exaggeration to claim the same situation existed for dementia but over the years, despite the availability of generally well-known definitions of the concept, dementia has meant all things to all men and women. As I sit through learned discussions on the minutiae of chemical, immunological and radiological technique I fear there is danger of forgetting the simple clinical formulation of dementia and with it the prospect of clear understanding of the concept. It will emerge in the book that what has been written, for instance, about alcoholic and metabolic dementias, has sometimes been the result of misapprehension and, in every sense, confusion about what the changes of dementia might be in those conditions. Rigorously applied and explicitly stated criteria were thought to be necessary for the schizophrenias and perhaps we must insist likewise for dementia.

Thirdly, one is always struck by the neglect of the subject of dementia.

Despite the torrent of statistical evidence and projections about the numbers of demented patients and the growing social importance of the syndrome, the subject still has not caught the popular imagination, medical or lay. I think a major obstacle to a serious study of dementia is the entrenched attitudes displayed by the traditional medical specialities and their preoccupations with demarcation disputes. A brief glance at the chapter headings will show a great variety of approaches to the subject. A speciality which refuses to acknowledge the value of scientific investigation or, on the other hand, washes its hands of the psychological and social aspects of the condition or refuses to soil them with the (for the present) often difficult management of hopelessly demented patients cannot hope to seriously contribute to advancement of knowledge. I suspect ideologies and doctrines of specialism are more important reasons for this neglect of dementia, though there may be something to be said for the claim that lack of concern might also owe a little to our unconscious fears of ageing and decrepitude, a point usually made by those of a metaphysical bent who can reach those parts of the soul that the rest of us cannot.

This book is an attempt to provide a critical account of the more important aspects of dementia as conceived at the present time. It aims to provide neurologists and psychiatrists in training and in preparation for the membership examinations, specialists in one or another area of investigation who wish to obtain a global overview of the syndrome, interested senior undergraduates, the hard-pressed general practitioner who might find himself in the vanguard of community care, nurses, social workers, occupational therapists and relatives of demented patients with an account which, it is hoped, will be manageably comprehensive. The works given for further reading are general and more accessible accounts for those who wish to know a little more, and those who want to pursue any subject at greater length have a set of references at the back of the book.

An incidental benefit in assembling these several conditions, which give the syndrome of dementia its rich variety, is the opportunity to describe their historical aspects. These stories are oft-told but are not always readily available. It will be clear that a historical perspective is vital to the understanding of dementia.

I make no apology for the presence of sections on social, ethical and pathographic aspects of the condition. It is plain that doctors will lead an increasingly sterile existence if they do not acknowledge those wider areas of life and living which might have a bearing on the course of illness and the practice of medicine. In any case, the points that have been made are of a very basic kind or are in the form of simple narrative. I hope they will serve as starting points for discussion, controversial if need be, and also encourage a more serious study of those individuals in public or artistic life who have become afflicted by dementia of one kind or another.

B MAHENDRA

Acknowledgements

I must thank Professor Michael Shepherd, Professor of Epidemiological Psychiatry at the Institute of Psychiatry, for providing me with a concise account of some aspects of the historical development of the concept of dementia. I have used this information in the historical chapter but I take sole responsibility for the views expressed therein.

The Librarian and staff of the St Bartholomew's Hospital Medical College Library at West Smithfield deserve my grateful thanks for the spendidly efficient way in which they obtained the literature I requested. I must thank, too, the Tate Library at Lambeth who loaned me several of the recorded issues and waited patiently for their return.

I have had helpful discussions with Gavin Brousson of the Alzheimer Disease Society, and COMBAT, the Association to Combat Huntington's chorea, made available some of their literature to me. May I take this opportunity to extend to both these voluntary organizations my very best wishes.

This book was written while I was on a grant given by the Wellcome Trust. Professor John Lumley of the Surgical Professorial Unit at St Bartholomew's Hospital directed the project and gave me every encouragement to keep writing.

1
Dementia: a brief history of the concept

The best way to suppose what may come is to remember what is past.
George Savile (1633–1695)

The concept of dementia that we know today, and which forms the subject-matter of this book, has evolved over many centuries. The problem has always been what to make of the term. Its derivation has not helped matters for 'dementia' corresponds to Latin *dementatus* – that is, out of one's mind, crazed, applicable to any and all abnormal, unusual, incomprehensible or bizarre behaviour.

In tracing the course of its distilled meaning – from the vantage point of over twenty centuries of hindsight – we shall see the term being adapted to suit conditions that were current in any given society. It is easy to understand that a concept now employed in most instances in relation to the elderly sick in the 20th century might not have had much meaning for the very different populations, patients and practitioners of the past.

For a start, living to be old was a distinctly unusual phenomenon in past centuries. Very few in the population survived to the senium, the period of life in which dementia becomes a calculable prospect rather than a chance occurrence. An estimate of those reaching the age of 65 in primitive society is around 3%; the life-span, on the average, of a subject in the Roman Empire was less than 30; an Englishman in 1700 could hope to live to a mean of 35 years; in 1840 the span of life had risen to 40–43 and in the 1980s it is 70–76, women living to the higher age.

In those early days, while the small numbers of the elderly would have shown the common cognitive changes associated with normal old age, only a minute proportion would have become demented in a modern sense. It is easy to see how the features of pathologic old age in the few would have been swamped by the relatively larger number of the elderly showing subtler physiological changes. This explanation would take care of growing old as an aetiological factor; the ancient role of such modern toxins as radiation,

1

transient viruses and metallic poisons we may never come to know.

This account of earlier approaches to senility and attitudes to old age owes much to George Rosen's excellent paper (1961). He quotes Cicero's essay on old age in the 2nd century BC. The major preoccupation in this age was the practice of mental hygiene. Poets and philosophers, at least, wondered if an active mental life might not forestall or postpone the decrepitude of old age. Cicero wrote:

> It is our duty to resist old age; to compensate for its defects by a watchful care; to fight against it as we would fight against disease. . . . Much greater care is is due to the mind and soul; for they, too, like lamps, grow dim with time, unless we keep them supplied with oil. . . . Intellectual activity gives buoyancy to the mind. . . . Old men retain their mental faculties, provided their interest and application continue . . . the aged remember everything that interests them. . . .   (Rosen, 1961)

This passage, which would not be out of place in a modern book on alternative health and mind care, also trails a familiar preoccupation of the next several centuries – mental hygiene for the prevention or postponement of old age. Cicero observes both the physical and mental effects of senility but there is no indication he attributed the changes to pathology. And the idea that intellectual activity could stave off the mental debilitation of the senium would have appeared quaint if some modern evidence did not lend support to it.

Celsus (30 BC–AD 50) probably first used the term 'dementia' in a medical context in the 1st century AD. In his encyclopaedia he is said to mention in passing that paralysis occurs in old age, but in his discussion of insanity there is no reference to old people. A century later the term 'senile dementia' itself seems to have been first used by Aretaeus, the physician of Cappadocia, but whether the concept had evolved to the point where it could be differentiated from the changes of normal old age is not known. Aretaeus commented on the mental decay of old age in discussing the differential diagnosis of a reversible form of excitement. He remarked this condition bore no resemblance to 'the dotage which is the calamity of old age . . . dotage commencing with old age never intermits, but accompanies the patient until death; while mania intermits, and with care ceases altogether' (Alexander, 1972). Mania was, of course, not necessarily the modern affective disorder but presumably any form of reversible mental illness with a component of excitement. This undoubtedly included delirium of organic causation.

In the 2nd century AD, when only a fraction of humanity was still destined to reach old age, Juvenal (AD 60–130) dealt with the subject with pessimism and bitterness in his tenth satire. This was the work that denounced the vanity of human wishes and warned of the tragedy of human hopes. Old age is ugly, deaf, blind, crippled by disease and deprived of reason.

> But worse than all bodily failing is the weakening mind which cannot remember names of slaves, nor the face of a friend he dined with last

evening, cannot remember the names of offspring begotten and reared. . . .

If you must pray for something, *orandum est ut sit mens sana in corpore sano*, which in a truncated form became a tag popularized by generations of schoolchildren.

Rosen then describes the work of Caelius Aurelianus a century later, who was influenced by Soranus of Ephesus, a physician in Rome at the time of the Emperors Trajan (AD 53–117) and Hadrian (AD 76–138). It appears that Caelius made several references to old age and mental illness and by this time, a full century after Celsus and Aretaeus, the pathological basis to some of the changes in the senium was being appreciated.

A couple of centuries later, in the 4th century AD, Oribasius, physician to the Emperor Julian, wrote of cerebral atrophy in his digest of medicine and surgery. This disease was thought to manifest itself in a loss of intellectual capacity and in weakness of movement. Oribasius tried to relate the condition to the ageing process and this was probably one of the earlier attempts to speculate as to aetiology of a more specific nature than mere old age.

By the 7th century AD the Byzantine physician, Paul of Aegina, was able to deal with the problems of loss of memory and reason in his writings. Rosen has said his discussion is obscure and it is uncertain as to whether senile dementia, feeblemindedness or aphasia were being dealt with. This is no reflection on Paul of Aegina as it was not until the 19th century that the distinction between the cognitive impairement due to dementia could be separated from that caused by mental handicap. The point to note, however, is that by this time loss of memory and reason had become subjects for legitimate study by physicians, as opposed to poets and philosophers. And as for the confusion between dementia and feeble-mindedness, it might well suggest that features, till then associated with the senium, were being observed in a younger age group.

As we have seen, states of excitement occasionally needed sorting out from dementia, but a more common cause of difficulty is likely to have been depression. Rosen notes that in the 9th century AD Rhazes the Persian physician mentions melancholy as an inevitable condition in the lives of old and decrepit persons. The Moslem writers of the Middle Ages seem to have had ideas similar to those of the Graeco-Romans on the nature of old age. The inevitable decrepitude and melancholic character of old age were commonplace ideas during the Renaissance period but the principal sources remained the ancient authors or mediaeval writers indebted to classical thought (Rosen, 1961).

Robert Burton (1577–1640), the author of *Anatomy of Melancholy*, observed that 'after seventy years all is trouble and sorrow'. He had views on the relationship between old age and melancholy too, saying that old age was 'natural to all . . . being cold and dry, and of the same quality as Melancholy is, must needs cause it, by diminution of spirits and substance. . . .'

Most people remember Shakespeare's (1564–1616) description of

> . . . lean and slippered pantaloon,
> With spectacles on nose and pouch on side
> His youthful hose, well saved, a world too wide
> For his shrunk shank; and his big manly voice,
> Turning again toward childish treble, pipes
> And whistles in his sound. Last scene of all
> That ends this strange eventful history,
> Is second childishness and mere oblivion,
> Sans teeth, sans eyes, sans taste, sans everything. (*As You Like It*)

but the bard has also to say:

> An old man is twice a child (*Hamlet)*

and

> You see me here, you gods, a poor old man,
> As full of grief as age; wretched in both! (*King Lear*)

which as the plot reveals is likely to have been something more than mere understandable reaction to a domestic dispute. Lear's senile peregrinations are well contrasted with the lunatic ravings of poor Tom O'Bedlam. The distinction between plain madness and senile decay is made clear and, like Burton, Shakespeare notes the association between cognitive and affective change.

We now move to the period between 1535 and 1860, the era covered by Hunter and Macalpine's excellent source book (1963). The authors include accounts of the involvement of several practitioners who involved themselves with cases of cognitive disorder. Philip Barrough (1560–1590), a licensed practitioner in Cambridge and author of a widely read textbook, seems to have drawn a distinction between loss of memory and loss of reason in cognitive disturbance.

> If reason be lost together with the memorie, then the affect is called *Fatuitas* or *stultitia* [that is] folishnes or doltishnes, and both these do come of one disposition, but that is more vehement wher both are hurte.

Richard Cosin, who lived in the later part of the sixteenth century, wrote an early account of the legal implications of insanity. *Inter alia* he considered six categories of 'wants of understanding and reason'. His 'dementia' refers to

> A passion of the minde, bereaving it of the light of understanding: Or . . . when a man's perceivance and understanding of all things is taken away, and may be englished distracted of wit, or being beside himself. (Hunter and Macalpine, 1963)

This, of course, is too wide-ranging and general to be a definition of mere cognitive change and suggests that while the features of the dementing

4

process could be recognized and described, the term 'dementia' was not necessarily appended to it. In fact, Cosin's other legal categories, *lethargie*–' . . . a notable forgetfulnes of all things almost, that hereto fore a man hath knowen . . . '; *delirium*–' . . . that weaknes of conceite and consideration, which we calle dotage: when a man, through age or infirmitie, falleth to be a childe again in discretion'; *stultitia*–' . . . that follie which is seen in such, as albeit they be but simple and grosse witted, yet are not to be accounted Idiotes, or Naturals . . . ', all contain elements of cognitive impairment amounting to dementia in its modern conception. The multiplicity of terms probably reflected the confusion in the ranks of the practitioners who were, as Cosin's interest in these matters suggests, not all medical men. Perhaps this attempt at a legal interpretation of the confused state of cognitive functioning in the 16th century was a foretaste of the legal profession's attempts to wrestle with the elusive concept of psychopathy four centuries later.

As Hunter and Macalpine note, early in the 17th century, Bedlam (Bethlem Hospital) was able to make its contribution to dementia. The Puritan divine, Thomas Adams, in his book *Mystical Bedlam OR The World of Mad-men* (1615) wrote of ' . . . some, that be hurt in both imagination and reason, and they necessarily therewithall doe lose their memories'. His other two categories refer to what in modern terms would be called delusions (erring in cogitation and reason) and hallucinations (problems with Phantasie and Imagination). These were subdivisions of the 'three internal senses or faculties . . . Imagination, Reason and Memorie'. They are clearly not mutually exclusive categories and one wonders how a demented patient with delusions and hallucinations might have fared. As melancholy in the sense of depressed affect was recognized and very likely given pride of place in any diagnostic hierarchy, it seems probable that problems of cognition continued to be understood and explained in terms of disordered affect, thought and perception except in the elderly when a primary disorder of higher functions could be invoked.

Hunter and Macalpine also include an account of one William Salmon (1644–1713), a practitioner who made his living apparently from patients turned away from St Bartholomew's Hospital, an early indication perhaps of attitudes to the less glamorous branches of the medical profession. He described a patient with senile dementia under the heading, 'Defects of Imagination, Reason and Memory in a Man superannuated' whom he diagnosed as 'not mad, or distracted like a man in Bedlam' but 'decayed in his Intellectuals'. He observed the early stages when such patients complain of depression and hypochondriacal symptoms and drew attention to the diagnostic triad of emotionality leading to involuntary laughing and crying associated particularly with arteriosclerotic dementia; loss of memory for recent events and perseveration (Hunter and Macalpine, 1963).

This brings us near the 18th century and the time is about right to embark on one of the more romantic stories in all medicine, the saga of general paresis. But before we, so to speak, take a break, it might be helpful to summarize what we have learned, with due warning that what we now say might well be conjecture and no more.

The earliest meaning of dementia is likely to have meant insane and seriously irrational behaviour. No distinction was presumably made between the normal and abnormal changes of old age until there were numbers of elderly in the population exhibiting this behaviour. At some point it must have been noted that the difficulties of some of the elderly were significantly different, and greater than that of the majority of their peers. Associated with this serious impairment in cognitive function was change in affect, mostly in the direction of depression, but cause and effect were probably beyond the understanding of observers. Whilst distinction could be drawn between the insanity of old age with a clear cognitive bias and the madness of younger patients with a predominant loss of reason and sense, there was almost certainly no concept of pre-senile dementia, no attempt apparently being made to distinguish between the cognitive failure of this group and those who were intellectually handicapped from a very early age.

AN INTERLUDE: THE STORY OF GENERAL PARESIS

Henry (1941) has given a straightforward account of the conventional view of the origins and discovery of general paresis. The evidence for the existence of general paresis prior to the early 19th century is thought to be inconclusive. Syphilis did not appear, at least in epidemic form, until after the return of Columbus from Haiti in 1493. Within a few years it had spread through Europe like a plague.

The recognition of general paresis as a separate disease entity was slow: conventional wisdom attributes this to Thomas Willis (1672). Willis wrote:

> In . . . cases . . . when, the brain being previously undisposed, they were visited with dullness of mind and forgetfulnes and then with stupidity and foolishness, they would afterwards fall into paralysis . . .

Hare (1959) has disputed the claims that Thomas Willis actually describes general paresis. Willis' passages in *De Anima Brutorum* are reviewed by Hare who believes much of the description would fit the case for arteriosclerotic dementia. He cites Robertson (1923), who had also expressed the view that it was 'much more likely that Willis refers to senile or arteriosclerotic dementia'.

After Willis one had to wait for more than a century for a communication which is possibly on the same subject, by John Haslam in 1798. Hare believes Haslam's claims to have observed general paresis to have been based on sounder evidence than Willis'. Haslam wrote:

> The paralytic affections are a more frequent cause of insanity than is believed. . . . As a rule the paralytics present disorders of motion, which are wholly independent of the mental disease . . . in the majority of patients memory is materially weakened. These patients, as a rule, fail to recognize their condition . . . [and] still maintain they are extremely strong and capable of the greatest deeds.   (Haslam, 1798)

However no satisfactory or unequivocal accounts of a disease corresponding to general paresis were given before those of the Parisian alienists in the early 19th century when anything from a sixth to a quarter of admissions to mental hospitals were for this illness (Hare, 1959). Esquirol in 1805 referred to the '. . . incurability of insanity complicated with paralysis', similar in prognostic hopelessness to the dementia of old age, but it had not occurred to Esquirol or anyone else that they were dealing with a separate and distinct disease entity (Henry, 1941).

In 1822 Bayle began presenting the conclusions to his clinical and pathological studies. He stated that the mental and physical symptoms are an expression of a single disease which is based upon a chronic inflammation of the meninges. Bayle was thus the first writer to affirm that general paresis was a disease entity characterized by disturbances of intellectual functions, by a variety of grandiose ideas peculiar to the disease and by progressive muscular inco-ordination and enfeeblement. He stated further that general paresis could not be considered as a complication of a mental illness and the symptoms did not occur as a part of any other form of mental illness (Henry, 1941).

Not deterred by all this, even as late as 1838, Esquirol continued to regard general paresis as a complication of various forms of mental disorder. (It is easy to see why clinicians cling to ideas like this. Cognitive disturbance was also probably considered for a long time as a complication of affective, melancholic or other 'mental' processes; perhaps it follows from the reductionist notion in medicine of trying to fit all symptomatology into a plausible, *single* diagnosis, most often a safe, well-established one. It is not simply the perversity of practitioners but a consequence of their upbringing.)

The specific aetiology for general paresis was not proposed until Esmarch suggested in 1857 that syphilis was the essential cause. Fournier had considered tabes dorsalis syphilitic in 1875 and in 1894 offered statistical evidence for the syphilitic origin of general paresis. But it was 1904 before a full description of the histopathological changes was given by Alzheimer.

In that same year Kraepelin had stated that 'syphilitic infection is essential for the later appearance of paresis'. Cerebrospinal fluid had been made practically available by Quinke's method in 1890 and when Wassermann's diagnostic test came into practice in 1906, an important link in the chain of evidence substantiating the theory of syphilitic origin of general paresis was forged. Further laboratory evidence was forthcoming with Lange's colloidal gold test discovered in 1912 (Henry, 1941).

Progress was being made on other fronts as well. In 1905 Schaudinn found the spirochaete in primary lesions and in 1913 *Treponema pallidum* was demonstrated in paretic brains by Noguchi and Moore. Ehrlich had discovered 'Salvarsan' (neoarsphenamine), the first of the modern pharmaceuticals, and this was pressed into service in 1910. In 1917 Wagner Von Jauregg was using fever therapy and, two world wars later, penicillin became the definitive treatment.

Hare (1959) has wondered why general paresis might have suddenly appeared on the firmament and then faded away only slightly less dramatically. From being a rare or non-existent disease it had become very prevalent in Paris in the early 19th century. From its origins in northern France the disease spread across Europe, then to America and later still to less highly industrialized countries. Hare believes there is evidence that during the subsequent 140 years the disease had shown gradual modifications in clinical form and a recent natural decline in prevalence, and that these changes are comparable with those that took place in the clinical course of syphilis during the years that followed the 15th century epidemic.

Hare further believes these points in the evidence will support the hypothesis that general paresis is due to a special 'neurotropic' strain of the syphilitic spirochaete, for they allow us to put forward the view that a mutation giving rise to the neurotropic strain occurred in northern Europe towards the end of the 18th century; that the spread of the mutant strain explains the time lapse before the disease was recognized in other countries; and that the new disease slowly changed in its prevalence and clinical manifestations (Hare, 1959).

Hare's thesis is an important one inasmuch as it considers the mutability of illness. If general paresis can arise relatively suddenly, so can other causes of dementia and their eclipse, for secular reasons, can be equally rapid. In a later interlude I shall discuss the recognition of Huntington's chorea, another illness that rose quickly to public prominence in the late 19th century after years of neglect. When one considers also the possibility of a kind of viral aetiology for Alzheimer's disease which has been mooted in a few quarters, one becomes cautious about commenting on diseases outside one's era. Not only concepts but diseases themselves may undergo change and break out of the Linnaean chains we like to impose upon them. Hare (1974) has further discussed the comings and goings of some other psychiatric illnesses including schizophrenia in a similar vein.

No account of any disorder with psychiatric manifestations in the 17th and 18th centuries would be complete without some mention of witchcraft, its alleged practitioners and the reaction of the public to them. There is little doubt now that the majority of persecuted witches were strange and solitary women given to various displays of eccentric behaviour. Some of them were old, and Rosen describes the last witch to be burnt in Scotland in 1722 as having been a very old woman. However, there seems little evidence that the psychiatric difficulties of these women were purely or mainly cognitive in nature. In fact, one would have thought that the pathetic mental and decrepit physical state of a truly demented woman would have evoked pity rather that the fear and loathing which seem to have fuelled much of the persecution. It would have been a different matter, though, if old women with cognitive defects had also exhibited physical 'stigmata' and the fate of female Huntington's choreics, as we shall see later, may well have been very different.

Modern psychiatry often traces its roots to Philippe Pinel (1745–1826), the humanitarian reformer of asylum practices who released the patients of the Bicetre and Salpetriere from their chains. He did not have much to say about dementia but uses the word 'demence' to designate one of the five classes of mental derangement and featuring 'the abolition of the thinking faculty'. However, he must have influenced his favourite, and most illustrious, pupil, Jean Etienne Dominique Esquirol (1772–1840), the very same as tried to make sense out of the signs of general paresis, who in 1838 published *Traite des Malades Mentales*, the fruit of 40 years' study of patients at the mental hospitals of Salpetriere and Charenton and in private practice. He defined dementia as a cerebral affection marked by a weakening of sensibility, understanding and will, and by the impairment of memory, reasoning and attention.

Esquirol distinguished three varieties of dementia: acute, chronic and senile. The acute variety could be caused by fever or haemorrhage and it was curable. The chronic form could be due to such factors as masturbation and drunkenness, or it could follow mania or epilepsy, and it was seldom cured. Clearly, Esquirol included a wide range of psychiatric disorders including delirium and functional illness in this conception. '*Demence senile*' is described as follows:

> Senile dementia results from the progress of age. There is . . . loss of sensibility along with . . . the faculty of understanding, before reaching an extreme state of decrepitude. Senile dementia . . . commences with feebleness of memory, particularly recent memory; attention . . . becomes impossible; the will is uncertain, the movements are slow . . . (Esquirol, 1838)

However, after this passage, which would seem unexceptionable as a modern description of dementia, Esquirol goes on to treat the origins of senile dementia in certain other cases. These were not rare instances, by any means. In fact Esquirol has said senile dementia 'began rather often' in this fashion. The passage that follows – which is an account of general excitement and hyperactivity, irritability, an increase in appetite for food, drink and sex – is clearly one that would sound like mania to modern ears and the 'dementia' that followed was very likely what we would call depression. Esquirol, then, was over-inclusive in his use of the term 'senile dementia' but his description of cognitive changes in some of those he considered demented in the senium brings him close to the modern conception.

Esquirol made a further contribution to our growing understanding of the concept. We have already seen that at least from the 7th century AD physicians had been confusing the cognitive impairment that follows a disturbance in the fully grown brain with that which arose in the undeveloped or partially developed brain. In other words, demented individuals were being confused with the intellectually subnormal. It is not clear why in the early 19th century attention should become focused on this difference. It may be, as so often is the case, that social pressures caused the minds of clinicians to be exercised. There was industrialization in the air, disturbing rustic life, and the subnormal who could be contained in villages, when the whole land was a village and life was uniformly simple, had now to be dealt with in new ways. The distinction between dementing intellectual impairment and subnormal intellectual deficit was no longer academic. It was also the heady years following the French Revolution and the other side of the coin to the mindless savagery of those times was a new humanitarian spirit that was abroad in the land. The treatment of the mentally ill and handicapped, who had no privileges worth speaking of, was no doubt under favourable review, not least by Pinel and Esquirol.

In 1838 Esquirol was able to sum up the difference between the demented and the mentally handicapped in an epigram: 'The dement is a man deprived of the possessions he once enjoyed, he is a rich man who has become poor. But the defective has been penniless and wretched all his life.' It could not have been put more succinctly.

James Cowles Prichard (1786–1848), physician and commissioner in Lunacy, described four stages of dementia that reflected its progression: impairment of recent memory, loss of reason, incomprehension and loss of instinctive action. He used the term 'Incoherency or Dementia' to denote a depression or a loss of the intellectual faculties. But views as to aetiology remained speculative. Prichard could add in 1842 that

> senile decay is occasionally the consequence of various disorders affecting the brain, such as long continued mania, or melancholia, or attack of apoplexy, or paralysis or severe and often repeated attacks of epilepsy or typhoid fevers in which the brain has been much affected. (Hunter and Macalpine, 1963)

Whilst the general idea seems to have been that organic change in the brain was needed to precipitate or sustain the cognitive impairment of old age, the early 19th-century practitioners were unwilling or unable still to separate the disorders of consciousness caused by acute injury and infection from the chronic course of dementia. Affective features could have been symptoms of organic disorder; also chronic, intractable depression could give a picture of persistent cognitive change, especially in that period a century before the availability of effective treatment, indistinguishable from dementia.

Conceptual advance was now not going to be rapid. Fifty years after Prichard, as the century turned, Tuke still managed to distinguish four types of dementia in the following fashion: primary or acute; secondary, which could follow mania or melancholia; senile; and paralytic. As with almost everyone on the continent in those early Kraepelinian days Tuke included cases of 'schizophrenia' under the heading of dementia.

In 1845 Wilhelm Griesinger's textbook on psychiatry had included a classification of 'apathetic dementia' under the general label of 'states of mental weakness'. Senile dementia was one example of apathetic dementia and thought to be due to disease of the cerebral arteries, a view that persisted until the time of Alzheimer. Griesinger was the quintessential exponent of the organic school of psychiatry. The phrase 'all mind diseases are brain diseases' has been attributed to him and he believed in the unitary nature of psychotic illness, i.e. mental illness is due to a single process and their manifestations are reflections of the stage and severity of the process.

A significant contribution to the mental pathology of old age was provided by Wille in 1873–1874. He endeavoured to clarify the aetio-logical, pathogenetic and pathologo-anatomical aspects of this area of investigation (Rosen, 1961). The major point of Wille's paper is the differential diagnosis of senile dementia from general paresis, the syphilitic aetiology of which would take another 20 years to establish. As for histopathology, we would have to wait till the first decade of the new century to be able to make the distinction between the two conditions. Wille also pointed out the importance of mild depressive reactions, presumably unrelated to organic change, and that these may end in suicide (Rosen, 1961).

Emil Kraepelin (1856–1926) was a student of Griesenger's who adopted the term 'organic dementias' for psychoses due to diseases of the central nervous system and thus narrowed the scope of the word dementia. Kraepelin's influential *Lehrbuch* in its 7th edition (1894) carried a well-defined clinico-pathological differentiation between senile dementia and psychoses with cerebral arteriosclerosis. Kreapelin's fame rests largely on his conception of what came to be known as schizophrenia. In 1898 he brought together various disparate conditions which had their onset in adolescence and early adult life and which he thought led inexorably to a demented state, and called this group of disorders *dementia praecox*. It became apparent that dementia was not inevitable in these patients and early in the new century 'dementia praecox' gave way to 'schizophrenia' or, more exactly, 'the schizophrenias'.

Also in 1898 Redlich reported miliary plaques in the brain in cases of senile cerebral atrophy associated with memory defects and mental confusion (Rosen, 1961). Gradually, histological and clinical studies began differentiating arteriosclerotic vascular disease from neurosyphilitic general paresis on the one hand, and from senile psychoses on the other.

Binswanger introduced the term 'pre-senile dementia' in 1898. Thus, at the turn of the century, the term dementia had become even more limited in usage. It was a condition that occurred in the senium and before; it was due to disease of the brain and thus clearly distinguishable from the neuroses that preoccupied Freud and the analysts in Vienna; and a reasonable distinction could be made between dementia due to general paresis, arteriosclerotic disease and a process in the senium. However, dementia had acquired the connotation of an irreversible mental disorder due to chronic brain disease. This view was challenged by some who felt dementia could be reversed and, in fact, made to disappear, but the term continued to be used for more than another half-century to refer to an irreversible and usually inexorably progressive organic mental disorder.

A BRIEF INTERLUDE: HUNTINGTON'S CHOREA

Huntington's chorea, Pick's disease, Alzheimer's disease and Creutzfeldt–Jakob disease constitute the classical quartet of pre-senile dementia. Huntington's chorea owes its name to George Huntington (1850–1916) who was a third-generation physician born into a community where several patients with the disorder attended his father's and grandfather's surgery. These patients were descendants of English stock who had emigrated to Connecticut from Suffolk.

11

In 1872 Huntington, who had qualified a year earlier, presented a paper entitled 'On chorea' in Ohio. The subject of his lecture was Sydenham's chorea but in concluding he drew attention to the familial chorea he had observed among patients in his father's practice.

Later in the same year his only written paper was published and he drew attention to 'three marked peculiarities' of the condition.

1. Its hereditary nature. 'When either or both the parents have shown manifestations of the disease . . . one or more of the offspring almost invariably suffer from the disease, if they live to adult age.'
2. 'The tendency to insanity, and sometimes that form of insanity which leads to suicide, is marked. . . . As the disease progresses, the mind becomes more or less impaired, in many amounting to insanity . . .'
3. 'Its third peculiarity is its coming on, at least as a grave disease, only in adult life. . . . While those who pass the fortieth year without symptoms of the disease are seldom attacked.' (Huntington, 1872)

The disease was called after Huntington but it is thought it can be traced back in history for several centuries. One study claimed to have found nearly 1000 cases, spanning twelve generations over 300 years, all of whom were believed to have been related to three emigrants from Suffolk who settled in New England in 1632. Another linked 173 French Canadian patients to a choreic woman who had emigrated from France to Montreal in 1645 (OHE, 1980).

The reason for the world's readiness to accept Huntington's description in 1872, and not acknowledge the disorder a couple of centuries before, may well be explained by the historical evidence that considerable hostility was directed against choreics. This does not seem surprising in view of the bizarre nature of both the chorea and the mental symptoms. In the 17th and 18th centuries, as we have seen, women who behaved oddly were pursued and persecuted, and patients with Huntington's chorea have the misfortune to be doubly eccentric. There must have been a conspiracy of silence, not least among the families and practitioners, for two centuries at least until the time was right for its 'discovery'.

Arnold Pick (1851–1924) was more interested in studying aphasia than in delineating another of the pre-senile dementias. In fact, doubt has been expressed if his account in 1892, based on the study of a patient's aphasia, was what we would call Pick's disease. Be that as it may, he had set the stage for Alzheimer's great contribution.

Alois Alzheimer (1864–1915) devoted his life to investigating the histopathology of dementia. When he started work two kinds of pathology of senile psychoses were acknowledged. In one kind all that was seen was generalized atrophy of the brain; in the other numerous healed infarcts could be seen.

In 1894, 10 years before his contribution to the histopathology of general paresis and 13 years before he made the findings which made his name, Alzheimer described the changes especially observed in arteriosclerotic atrophy of the brain. These were patients in their fifth and sixth decades who presented with apoplexy, paralysis, a labile affect, regression of reasoning and a loss of memory. Histologically, he found severe arteriosclerotic changes in the vessels of the brain and associated tissue degeneration. Changes were also noted in the heart and the kidneys; the changes in the brain blood vessels extended to the smallest branches, and around the vessels the naked eye could detect wide areas filled with liquid, especially around the basal ganglia and the internal capsule. Focal softening of the brain was another feature. Alzheimer also gave a description of the clinical features corresponding to the pathology he saw. It tallies closely with what we might call vascular or arteriosclerotic dementia.

The recognition of what came to be known as Alzheimer's disease was made possible by new histological techniques that utilized silver impregnation to stain cellular elements of the brain. In this way senile plaques were recognized as early as 1892, but the stains used then chiefly affected glial elements. In 1903 Bielschowsky modified the technique of staining so that neurones could be impregnated and studied for the first time.

Certain cases of pre-senile dementia and macroscopic brain atrophy revealed senile plaques and neurofibrillary changes consisting of thick argentophilic fibrils within the cytoplasm. Alzheimer had not been the first to describe senile plaques but recognized that plaques in large numbers might be abnormal; neurofibrillary tangles he considered specific for dementia.

In 1907 Alzheimer reported on a 51-year-old woman who presented with morbid jealousy, loss of memory, capricious behaviour, spatial and temporal disorientation, persecutory ideas and speech difficulties. The focal symptoms were always mild but the dementia progressed and she was dead within 5 years. To the naked eye her brain appeared atrophied without obvious lesions on the surface, though the larger vessels seemed atherosclerosed. Microscopically, inside cells, numerous thick fibrils taking on silver stain were found. Up to a third of cells had a metabolic product deposited in the cell, and scattered throughout the cortex, especially in the upper layers, were found numerous foci due to the deposition of a peculiar substance. There was no infiltration of the blood vessels (Alzheimer, 1907–translated 1969).

It is only fair to point out that the clinical features described by Alzheimer in his famous patient will not always now be considered typical of what we would call Alzheimer's disease. But in 1907 Kraepelin suggested this curious disease be called after Alzheimer and in the next 5 years some 50 papers had been published on the subject. The cases in the literature were characterized by early age of onset; symptoms of aphasia, apraxia and agnosia; and the pathologically distinctive neurofibrillary tangles. Alzheimer was convinced of a distinction from arteriosclerosis and ageing but Kraepelin was less certain, finding that the disease could arise in quite young patients. In 1910 he contented himself by saying, 'The clinical significance of Alzheimer's disease is at present still uncertain.'

Initially the diagnosis of Alzheimer's disease was dependent upon both clinical and pathological characteristics but the specificity of senile plaque was already being questioned. The specificity of the other element in the histopathological diagnosis, the neurofibrillary tangle, also became uncertain when it was found outside dementing illness, as in amyotrophic lateral sclerosis and post-viral Parkinson's disease. Soon it became known that large numbers of normal people in the senium had some senile plaques and neurofibrillary tangles. In 1936 Jervis and Soltz advised that only clinical criteria would suffice for a diagnosis of Alzheimer's disease.

The question had to be answered if the separation of dementia before and after the age of 65 had any validity, if senile and pre-senile dementia had distinction beyond age. As will be seen later, the answer cannot still be unequivocally given. Cerebral blood flow measurements became available after 1945 and it seemed blood flow was diminished in dementia; a revival of the theory of the aetiological importance of a lack of blood in dementia was short-lived, however, as it became clear that diminished blood flow was likely to follow cerebral atrophy and dementia rather than be a cause of them.

By now, dementia had come to be seen as an irreversible mental disorder due to chronic brain disease. A distinction was being drawn between this and delirium, which is a reversible mental disorder due to acute brain disease. As late as 1960 the standard British text on clinical psychiatry could still speak of dementia as a chronic, irreversible and untreatable condition. As ever, the concepts of an illness had to reflect the environment in which the illness had to be diagnosed and treated. Investigation and management of systemic and functional psychiatric illness had to advance before dementia could be conceived as being treatable and reversible, even then only in a minority of cases.

Accordingly, in the 1960s, several writers in England and Germany called for a revision of the concept and emphasized that irreversibility should not be viewed as an essential feature of dementia. It became increasingly clear that identical clinical features of intellectual deterioration could be caused both by irreversible cerebral diseases and by more or less reversible ones. This is the situation that prevails today, and is the subject of chapter 2.

A CODA: CREUTZFELDT–JAKOB DISEASE

The original descriptions were by Creutzfeldt in 1920 and Jakob in 1921, of cases of dementia with pyramidal and extrapyramidal signs. Creutzfeldt's case is now excluded from the group of spongiform encephalopathies, among which the disease is classified. Jakob's original five slides were reviewed more than 50 years after they were made by Masters and Gajdusek (1982) who feel two of Jakob's five cases had the type of changes which make them fall within present-day diagnostic criteria for spongiform encephalopathy.

The disease, which is occasionally familial, is rare and the neuropathological findings are those of a degenerative disease of the nervous system, in which there is a tendency for nerve cells to vacuolate and to die, for astrocytes to swell and to proliferate, and for the grey matter to reflect the neuronal and glial changes by developing a spongy look (Corsellis, 1979). The histological picture is neither reminiscent of an inflammatory reaction nor does it point to the possibility of an infection.

Masters and Gajdusek believe the two 'positive' cases represent the earliest proven examples of subacute spongiform encephalopathy. Matters might have rested there and Creutzfeldt–Jakob disease would have remained a largely historical curiosity if Gajdusek and Zigas (1957) had not identified the condition called Kuru, a degenerative disease of the central nervous system with a genetic bias leading to cerebellar ataxia, in certain tribes in the Eastern Highlands of Papua-New Guinea. Hadlow (1959) thought Kuru resembled a disease in sheep called scrapie, which is transmissible from sheep to sheep as well as from sheep to goats and mink by the injection of 'infected' brain tissue. Following this up, Gajdusek discovered that brain tissue from a dead Kuru patient could infect a chimpanzee via its brain. Observations like this soon led to the suspicion that the spread of Kuru was at least partly through abraded skin during ritual cannibalism (Corsellis, 1979).

Very soon after Hadlow's observations a relationship between Kuru and Creutzfeldt–Jakob disease began to be suspected, and could be confirmed with reasonable certainty when the infected biopsy tissue from a Creutz-feldt–Jakob patient was successfully transmitted to a chimpanzee. At autopsy the animal's brain showed the histological features which are common to scrapie, Kuru and Creutzfeldt–Jakob disease. By 1968, therefore, the transmissible nature of Creutzfeldt–Jakob disease had been established and it was placed within the group of 'transmissible subacute spongiform encephalopathies' due, it is thought, to an unconventional group of 'slow viruses'. In 1974 a case was reported of Creutzfeldt–Jakob disease which had arisen and run to a fatal conclusion after the patient had received a corneal graft from a donor who suffered from the disease.

A CHRONOLOGY OF DEMENTIA

1st century AD	— First medical use of the term 'dementia' by Celsus (30 BC–AD 50). Up to then poets had lamented the ravages of age on the mind.
2nd century AD	— Aretaeus, the Physician of Cappadocia, uses the term 'senile dementia' but may well have described changes of senescence.
	— A pathological basis to some of the difficulties of old age may have been considered by Caelius Aurelianus.
7th century AD	— Paul of Aegina, a Byzantine physician, is writing about loss of memory and reason, but George Rosen thought he might have been confusing dementia and feeblemindedness.
9th century AD	— Rhazes, the Persian physician, refers to the association between age and decrepitude and melancholy.

15

To 16th century AD — Columbus had returned from the New World in 1493, bringing syphilis with him.

— The inevitability of decrepitude and melancholy became commonplace ideas. Shakespeare (1564–1616) makes reference to this in one of his best-known passages and to the distinction between senile insanity and ordinary madness in *King Lear*. Not surprisingly, perhaps, it is considered one of his more horrifying works.

16th century AD — Loss of memory is being distinguished from loss of reason but a combination is thought to lead to a more serious state.

— 'Dementia' still does not mean what we mean, and terms like lethargie, delirium and stultitia convey a more modern flavour.

17th century AD — Problems of reason and memory were being seen in the same light as delusions and hallucinations but cognitive impairment was probably still explained in terms of change of affect.

— In 1672 Thomas Willis published *De Anima Brutorum*. The first descriptions of general paresis are often traced to this work but it has been said they might have described senile or arteriosclerotic dementia.

— Persecution of witches a feature. Little evidence that demented women, unless they showed physical characteristics like chorea, were preferentially persecuted.

18th century AD — Witches still at risk.

— In 1798 Haslam describes conditions which might make his, rather than Willis', the pioneering British observations on general paresis.

— The French Revolution. Diseased, as opposed to titled heads, could look forward to a new deal including release from chains in psychiatric hospitals and more humane treatment generally.

19th century AD — In 1822 Bayle provides a description which establishes general paresis as a distinct entity.

— In 1838 Esquirol makes a distinction between the mentally ill and the mentally subnormal.

— In 1845 Griesinger thinks senile dementia might be due to disease of the cerebral arteries.

- In 1857 Esmarch suggests syphilis might be the cause of general paresis.

- In 1872 George Huntington describes cases of hereditary chorea which was regularly seen in his father's and grandfather's surgeries before him.

- In 1892 Arnold Pick describes his eponymous case of dementia with aphasia.

- In 1894 Emil Kraepelin distinguishes between senile and arteriosclerotic dementia, as does Alzheimer.

- In 1898 Kraepelin proposes his concept of *dementia praecox* which is held to be partially mistaken in the next decade.

- In 1898 Binswanger suggests the adjective 'presenile'.

20th century AD
- In 1904 Alzheimer describes the histopathology of general paresis.

- In 1905 Schaudinn discovers the spirochaete in the primary syphilitic lesion.

- In 1907 Alzheimer describes the case of the 51-year-old woman with dementia and the distinctive neuropathology which would make him famous.

- In 1913 Noguchi and Moore find the spirochaete in paretic brains.

- In 1920 Creutzfeldt, and in 1921 Jakob, describe cases of dementia with pyramidal and extrapyramidal signs. Creutzfeldt's case is not now considered to be spongiform encephalopathy but Creutzfeldt–Jakob disease is given to the world.

- In 1957 Kuru is identified in some cannibals in the Eastern Highlands of Papua-New Guinea.

- 1960 and the standard British psychiatric textbook still considers dementia to be chronic and irreversible; the reversibility of normal pressure hydrocephalus, described in 1965, and progress in the investigation and treatment of growing numbers of systemic disorders, helps change this view.

- In 1968 the transmissible nature of Creutzfeldt–Jakob disease, Kuru and scrapie, which are related to one another, is established.

Further reading

(A full list of references is given at the end of the book)

Alexander, D.A. (1972). 'Senile dementia': a changing perspective. *Br. J. Psychiatry*, **121**, 207–214

Corsellis, J.A.N. (1979). On the transmission of dementia. A personal view of the slow virus problem. *Br. J. Psychiatry*, **134**, 553–559

Hare, E.H. (1959). The origin and spread of dementia paralytica. *J. Ment. Sci.*, **105**, 594–626

Henry, G.W. (1941). Organic mental diseases. In Zilboorg, G. and Henry, G.W. (eds) *A History of Medical Psychology*. (New York: W.W. Norton)

Hunter, R. and Macalpine, I. (1963). *Three Hundred Years of Psychiatry, 1535–1860*. (London: Oxford University Press)

Office of Health Economics (1980). *Huntington's Chorea*. (London)

Rosen, G. (1961). Cross cultural and historical approaches. In Hoch, P.H. and Zubin, J. (eds) *Psychopathology of Ageing*. (New York: Grune and Stratton)

Talbott, J.H. (1970). Alois Alzheimer. In *A Biographical History of Medicine*. (New York: Grune and Stratton)

2
Dementia: general considerations

A mind quite vacant is a mind distressed.

William Cowper (1731–1806)

We have seen traced in general terms in the previous chapter the evolution of a kind of understanding of the meaning of the term dementia. As we have seen, this modern understanding has been arrived at not only by observations and descriptions of cognitive disturbance of a serious and clearly pathological kind in the senium and before, but by those conditions like general paresis, Huntington's chorea and Creutzfeldt–Jakob disease, which have striking associated neurological features and were initially studied as much for these as for the disorders of higher function that are seen with them.

Whilst, therefore, the term dementia may have meant many things to many men over many centuries, a consensus definition in keeping with the knowledge we have about dementia in the present day is now accepted in practice.

Three definitions made in the past decade or so reflect this consensus.

(1) Dementia is an acquired global impairment of intellect, memory and personality but without impairment of consciousness (Lishman, 1978).

(2) Dementia is the global impairment of higher cortical functions including memory, the capacity to solve the problems of day-to-day living, the performance of learned perceptuo-motor skills, the correct use of social skills and control of emotional reactions, in the absence of gross clouding of consciousness. The condition is often irreversible and progressive (Report of the Royal College of Physicians by the College Committee on Geriatrics, 1981).

(3) The third edition of the American Psychiatric Association Diagnostic

19

and Statistical Manual (DSM III, 1978) lists the following criteria for the diagnosis of dementia:

(i)   A deterioration of previously acquired intellectual abilities of sufficient severity to interfere with social or occupational functioning.
(ii) Memory impairment.
(iii) At least one of the following: (a) impairment of abstract thinking; (b) impairment in judgement or impulse control; (c) personality change.
(iv) Failure to meet the criteria for 'intoxication' or 'delirium', although these may be superimposed.
(v)   Either of the following: (a) evidence from physical examination, laboratory tests, or history of a specific organic factor judged to be causally related to the disturbance; or (b) in the absence of such evidence, the assumption of the existence of an organic factor necessary for the development of the syndrome.

This last item is a somewhat controversial criterion and is taken up later.

A very clinical concept

The first point to be made is that the definitions given, the last contentious paragraph of DSM III excepted, are entirely in regard to clinical considerations. The features noted are symptoms and signs. Their assessment is by a clinician and it is he who decides upon the diagnosis. It will be recalled that attempts have been made, for instance, by using pneumencephalography and, in more recent years, computerized tomography, to make an assessment and, indeed in some instances, a diagnosis of dementia. This must have been due to a misunderstanding of the concept of dementia. Nowhere in the definitions is cerebral atrophy or ventricular enlargement (two of the more common features looked for in neuroradiological assessment) mentioned as components of the dementia syndrome. No radiological feature is established to be related to the cardinal features of dementia, intellectual deterioration, memory deficit and personality disorganization. The place of radiology is a more limited one, and, at present, limited largely to an investigation of the causes of dementia, and is discussed in Chapter 7. The role of the electroencephalograph, in so far as it may be used as a measure of severity of dementia, is slightly and subtly different but in essence similar – EEG changes do not figure in the definition of dementia and have only limited correlation with the cardinal features of the syndrome, as we shall see in Chapter 5.

The psychologist is in a somewhat different position. Normally his first involvement with a patient suspected of being demented is in order to confirm the symptoms of intellectual deterioration, memory deficit and, more unusually, personality change detected on clinical examination. If, however, the psychologist involves himself by taking an informed history in the usual manner instead of limiting himself to measuring deficit and allocating numbers, he is in a good position to make the diagnosis because what he will be concerning himself with will be elements in the definition of the concept.

20

The pathologist cannot make the diagnosis of the syndrome, as opposed to its causes, by pathological study alone. Dementia is to do with failing cognitive function and the disorders of behaviour which follow, and is not solely a matter of plaques, neurofibrillary tangles and infarctions. However, if a neuropathologist can make a diagnosis of, say, Alzheimer's disease on histopathology with the aid of defined criteria he may have a certain expectation that his patient has, or had, dementia, but this is in terms of probability. It is well established, of course, that several of the histological features of Alzheimer's disease are found to a lesser extent, in quantitative terms, in normal old age and in some non-dementing states and the relationship between the pathological changes of Alzheimer's disease and the clinical syndrome of dementia need not be invariable.

A concept for our time

We must hasten to stress that the concept of dementia we have employed is in terms of present knowledge and usage. We have previously, in the last chapter, seen the concept evolving, and it is perfectly possible that with advances in knowledge the concept and diagnostic criteria will change. Advances in histopathology and neurochemistry are discussed in Chapter 8. If the diagnosis of dementia is to be made in terms of, say, the presence or absence of a quantity of a chemical substance in the brain or blood, the pathologist and histochemist will come into their own. If, on the other hand, as will be seen in Chapter 7, the diagnosis comes to be seen in terms of radio-absorption densities of brain tissue, the neuroradiologist obviously will become the key diagnostician. But, at present, within the confines of our concept, only the clinician (and this includes the technical specialist who is prepared to play clinician) is able to make a valid diagnosis of dementia.

The idea of change in the clinical state in dementia is an important one. The definition from the Royal College of Physicians (1981) has that dementia '. . . is *often* irreversible and progressive' (author's emphasis). This is a relatively recent idea, current for the past decade or so. As late as 1960 the standard British work on clinical psychiatry (Mayer-Gross *et al.*, 1960) defined dementia as an 'irreversible decline in mental functions'. This is now not thought to be invariable and an important group of dementias, called the secondary dementias and discussed at length in Chapter 3, is now recognized. They may, depending on the stringency with which the definition of dementia is applied, the degree of investigatory enthusiasm shown, the age of the patients investigated and the speciality of the institution (medical, neurological or psychiatric) concerned, contribute anything up to 25% of all cases of dementia. Their recognition has banished the investigatory and therapeutic nihilism that plagued the study of dementia and has helped bring about this salutary change in the concept.

If reversal of the dementing process is acknowledged, the question of the time over which changes can occur must be considered. Note of the duration of the process is not usually made in definitions of dementia but it is implicit in the approach to dementia. Virtually no clinician will make the diagnosis if the process has lasted less than several weeks and one author (Hughes, 1978) maintains a period of 6 months or more of a symptomatic

21

state is required before a safe diagnosis can be made. This is caution that is designed to minimize false-positive diagnosis. A glance at the definitions of dementia reminds us how vaguely general the descriptions of cognitive and behavioural change are. To be mildly facetious, if only to prevent the degeneration of the concept of dementia into absurdity, one can point out that if the idea of sustained change is not appreciated all kinds of conditions which show psychic phenomena but are only nominally medical – like drunkenness, the state of hangover and premenstrual tension – might well be accommodated within the meaning of the definition.

The idea of reversibility also brings home to us the prospect of changing clinical states. If a patient presents with the main features of dementia, viz. intellectual deterioration, memory deficit and personality change, but on follow-up loses one or all of these and is left with features of, say, depression or indeed recovers fully, has he or hasn't he got dementia? More to the point, did he have dementia? A brief case history of a 62-year-old man who presented with features of dementia but also had depression illustrates the problem rather well. Now, his depression could have been a symptom of his dementia or it could have been the cause of the dementing picture, a state of affairs which has been called 'pseudo-dementia' and which is now recognized to be an important 'secondary' or 'treatable' cause of dementia. A diagnosis of dementia was made and he was followed up a year later. He was found to be unchanged clinically. The diagnosis could very easily have been upheld without dissent if his son had not been interviewed a second time. It transpired that in the year past the patient had been treated with tricyclic antidepressant medication and in fact had made a full recovery. He had subsequently stopped taking his (now) prophylactic medication and had had a relapse of his depressive illness. Not surprisingly, the course of his illness approximated to the course in the previous year. He could well have gone on to having an annual bout of depressive illness and if his interim state had not been taken into account the more complex nature of his diagnostic formulation would not have been known. The real danger in this case was, of course, that at the annual assessment the doctor might have been convinced of the inefficacy of the antidepressant medication, stopped it altogether and started managing the patient as an average, admittedly hopeless, case of idiopathic dementia.

This case history also illustrates two further points about dementia which will now be taken in turn. The first is to ask ourselves whether or not dementia is a solely descriptive state. From the definitions it seems it clearly is. There is no aetiological consideration when one establishes the presence or absence of the condition. Yet, in the previous paragraph, it was hinted that a distinction is sometimes made between 'true' dementia and 'pseudo'-dementia. This is not a logical state of affairs in terms of the definition of dementia we now use, and is in fact a throwback to the days when dementia had to be seen to be irreversible before it could be called thus. It can now be argued that a case such as the one that was illustrated is an example of 'secondary' dementia and can with advantage be treated with others of a similar description. This theme is further pursued in Chapter 3.

The other point that emerged from the case illustrated was the importance of the history or, to put it another way, an account of the cause of the illness. If one looks again at the definitions of dementia, one is struck by the fact that though intellectual and mnesic ability is stressed in the here and now, their importance to the clinical picture is the change they have undergone. It is intellectual *deterioration* and memory *deficit*, a change from a previous state, that are required. It stands to reason that a man losing his intellect and memory, whether on a permanent or temporary basis, is not likely to give an accurate account of the course of his difficulties. It is therefore of the most vital importance that an independent history be obtained, and it may be taken as axiomatic that a diagnosis of dementia cannot be made unless an assessment can be made of the previous state of the patient or the onset and course of the symptoms. It need hardly be added that neither a physical nor mental state examination, nor any investigation, is likely to throw light on these matters. A few brief general points regarding the assessment of the demented patient are made at the end of this chapter, and a more detailed plan is given in the Appendix.

Another point to be made is that dementia is an *acquired* condition. There is no entity corresponding to congenital dementia. Yet, cognitive and behavioural impairment is seen in individuals before the age of 16 or so, the age after which dementia can be diagnosed. This state is, of course, usually called mental subnormality or handicap. We have seen how Esquirol made the distinction between dementia and amentia in 1838 and there was speculation as to why it had taken that long to make the distinction. It is an important difference, nonetheless. Subnormality is usually suspected and diagnosed on social and educational grounds, and the condition is almost invariably noted in childhood. For historical reasons the management of subnormality has devolved upon the medical profession yet the problems of the management of the subnormal – apart from being a life-long consideration – are social, legal and educational. Three-quarters of those who are subnormal have mild or 'subcultural' handicap, and a very large proportion of the subnormal have no discernible medical feature to their condition. The very obvious feature of dementia is the medical nature of the condition. The question of education or re-training does not arise with demented patients as it does with the subnormal, and much of the management of dementia at present involves providing relatively short-term care. The majority of dements are over 65 and much of their life has been spent. The distinction between the two states is a clear and very necessary one though we have had it only for the past 150 years. The intriguing connection between older Down's syndrome patients' brains and Alzheimer disease brains is considered in a later chapter.

It follows also from the definitions that dementia is a global condition. This might seem an obvious remark to make concerning a condition which involves primarily the intellect, memory and personality. The reason for stressing this is that a collection of focal deficits, however severe, does not amount to dementia. Also, intellect, memory or personality can be individually affected. In Korsakoff's syndrome there can be a devastating immediate and short-term memory deficit but since this is the only component of the dementia syndrome present, Korsakoff's syndrome is clearly not dementia though much patience and skill may be required to rule out intellectual deficit. In a stroke affecting one or the other cerebral hemispheres considerable damage may be done to verbal or performance intelligence, yet if the other elements in the definition of dementia are not found with this it does not amount to dementia. Personality change may be found in functional psychiatric conditions, most characteristically in schizophrenia, but intellect and memory are usually preserved, though not invariably, as we shall see when 'pseudo-dementia' is discussed.

Distinction from other cognitive disorders

There is no differential diagnosis of dementia. As with other descriptive states such as fever or anaemia, the differential diagnosis is between the causes of dementia, which is the subject of Chapter 3. However, distinction is possible, and necessary, between dementia and other states of disordered cognition.

We have seen that it is important to be able to distinguish between focal deficits and dementia. One cause of difficulty is aphasia. In dementia speech difficulties can be placed in the context of impairment of cognitive features generally. It is a progressive and, generally, relatively late feature. Quite apart from difficulties in general behaviour, non-verbal activity is also affected.

In contrast, the patient with a focal deficit has difficulty generally only with behaviour related to language. The onset in the more usual type of focal impairment is sudden, as with cerebrovascular disease, and may be the only disturbance of higher functioning although characteristic changes in motor, sensory and reflex activity and visual field defects would normally be expected to assist in the localization. The speech of a person with jargon aphasia, which results from lesions in Wernicke's area, may sound like demented speech – voluble, fluent, effortless and articulate but meaningless. Elements of normal speech may be amusingly combined to form nonsense words or neologisms and substitution of words that have similar sounds or similar meanings may occur (Ropper, 1979).

The absence of gross clouding of consciousness is a vital element in the definition of dementia, for cognitive functions of all kinds are disturbed in states of disordered consciousness, from toxic confusion to coma. A drunken man or a delirious one is quite clearly affected in terms of intellect, memory, personality and general behaviour. Equally clearly they cannot be called demented unless one wishes to confuse the concept. The only exception is in the late, terminal stages of dementia when a marked disorientation can supervene. But by then the history is quite clear. It is, of course, possible for a demented patient, like anyone else, to acquire a condition which leads to toxic confusion. The logical thing to do in these conditions is to wait for the clouding to disperse before making an assessment of the dementia.

This distinction is an important one and failure to observe it can only help debase the concept of dementia. Yet, in an otherwise valuable review, Ropper (1979) was led to observe that 'confusion . . . is a major component of the dementia syndrome, although it can also result from a toxic or metabolic encephalopathy'. It is believed that a failure to observe this distinction has led to the long lists of causes of treatable dementias which festoon textbooks. It is now thought likely that a large number of drugs and metabolic and endocrine encephalopathies lead to 'confusions' and cognitive changes involving clouding of consciousness rather than dementia. As Roth (1982) observes,

> ... the brain is well insulated from the adverse metabolic effects of most forms of extra-cerebral disease. If chronic respiratory, cardiovascular, hepatic and renal disease cause any psychiatric complication they almost invariably give rise to a sub-acute, fluctuating clouded or delirious state. The same statement can be made for many cases of pernicious anaemia and other toxic and deficiency diseases that figure in lists of aetiological causes of dementia. However, such causes may potentiate an associated dementia which remains after these disorders have been treated.

On an earlier occasion he had said (Roth, 1980)

> in practice ... states of disturbed consciousness arising without warning are virtually never prodromal features of progressive cerebral disease unless there is concomitant evidence for a focal neurological lesion.

The details which help in making this distinction between dementia and clouding of consciousness are tabulated (Table 2.1).

A state which illustrates an affection of a single element of the dementia syndrome is the dysmnesic syndrome. It often begins with clouding of consciousness and delirium and when this has subsided a pure impairment of short-term memory may be a sequel. Though classically associated with the Wernicke–Korsakoff syndrome, it is now believed to arise in several other conditions including head injury and cerebrovascular disease. As we have seen before, skilled and patient examination of these patients reveals preserved intellectual functioning, which is a point of distinction from the demented patient who might display a similar disorder of memory. Also, the personality in patients with the dysmnesic syndrome is seen, with careful observation, to be reasonably well preserved and does not undergo the deterioration and disorganization that the demented patient's does.

GENERAL CLINICAL FEATURES OF DEMENTIA

Lishman (1978) and Roth (1980) have given detailed descriptions of the early and more general features of the demented patient.

The onset is usually insidious but the features of disturbed cognitive state do not bring the patient to the doctor. This is often brought about because of some intercurrent illness or for some social reason, such as the loss of a spouse or a change of dwelling. Occasionally some seriously disturbing or

Table 2.1   Distinguishing dementia from clouded consciousness (after several authors)

Dementia	*Clouding of consciousness*
1. Women predominate in the commoner dementias.	1. Men predominate 2 : 1.
2. Long duration of state, measured in months or years.	2. Short duration, lasting days or weeks.
3. Intervals of normal functioning rare and short-lived.	3. Marked variability of degree of mental impairment with lucid intervals.
4. Severe impairment of intellectual activity at all times.	4. Intellectual ability unimpaired, especially during lucid intervals.
5. Memory failure is both short-term and remote.	5. Memory impairment short-term.
6. Deteriorated and disorganized personality.	6. Intact personality.
7. A negative and dull disorientation in keeping with ideational poverty.	7. Active and creative disorientation often shown as imaginative confabulation.
8. Vague, fleeting hallucinations.	8. Marked, florid hallucinations, usually visual and terrifying. Visual misinterpretation prominent.
9. Random and vague persecutory ideas and delusions.	9. Acute, prominent persecutory ideas and delusions.
10. Apathetic and flat emotions.	10. Fear and perplexity well marked.

dangerous behaviour such as wandering away, becoming abusive or assaultive, being involved in, or thought liable to, accidents to themselves or others, or some criminal misdemeanour, might bring them to the attention of the medical or social services.

As will be seen in the section on early dementia, one of the difficulties is assessing the onset of the condition. The early manifestations are attributed to normal ageing in which both difficulties with memory and an exaggeration of traits of personality, often the less desirable ones such as self-centredness and rigidity, might be noted.

The earliest feature is usually an impairment of recent memory. This difficulty is not confined to the short term but progresses to involve earlier and more remote events. As Roth (1980) states, much has been made of the disturbance of short-term memory being somehow characteristic or even pathognomonic of the dementing condition, but the evidence is against this. The average patient with dementia is seen to have a more widespread disorder of memory.

Roth shows that in problems of intellectual functioning, abstract thought is particularly vulnerable. The patient is unable to discern common themes or essential differences. He finds new situations confusing and his ideas are

26

meagre. The lack of grasp leads to false ideas which may become delusional but evidence of their falsehood cannot be understood (Roth, 1980).

The classic description of personality change in dementia is one of 'coarsening' of the character. Often the less attractive characteristics such as rudeness, tactlessness, thoughtlessness and selfishness, already present in the premorbid state, may become accentuated in the early stages. These may only be socially disadvantageous but involvement with the law might come about through inappropriate sexual behaviour or thieving, conduct which is invariably out of character. Emotional changes are common in the early stages and significant depression, which can delay the diagnosis, may be present; elation or a manic-affect is less common. As the dementia progresses these 'positive' effects give way to an emotional blunting or apathy and the patient, deprived of both the intellectual and emotional contents of his being, becomes a human shell in the terminal stages. He is not spared physically, either, and in the later stages becomes shrunken and shrivelled and walks with a slow, shuffling gait.

Wells (1979) has listed some features which might be seen in the early stages of dementia – expression of too much satisfaction from trivial accomplishments; struggling too hard to perform at a level that would previously have required little effort; referring to notes, guides and calendars too freely; expressing disinterest on a topic and stating that sons or daughters keep up with it, and indicating a subsequent return to a question but neglecting to return. It is easy to see how difficult in practice it might be to distinguish these features from the norm for any given patient, and in any case many of these features come to light only with hindsight.

Neurological signs

No neurological sign is pathognomonic or characteristic of dementia and they do not figure in the definition of dementia. However, dementia is due, in the vast majority of instances, to serious and prolonged diseases of the brain, and it is to be expected that a few signs will be associated with it. A number of 'reflexes' fall into this category, though they may also be found in many other diffuse cerebral diseases, and have been described by Ropper (1979).

In the *grasp reflex*, contact with the patient's palm elicits grasping. The demented patient's frequent clutching and picking at the bedsheets is a reflection of this. In the tonic foot *response* the toes turn downwards when the sole is stimulated by non-painful pressure. Sucking, snouting, mouthing, puckering and rooting are all variations of the primitive response to stroking or percussing the oral region. The *palmomental reflex* which is seldom seen in normal adults increases with age and is common in dementia.

In addition to these reflexes a number of other signs are seen in dementia. Motor impersistence, or the inability to maintain a simple posture, such as keeping the eyes closed or protruding the tongue, is common in dementia as well as with lesions of the right parietal lobe. Perseverance, the converse of impersistence, may also be seen.

Ropper also describes the characteristic gait in dementia, *marche a petits*

27

pas, in which the person has a flexed stance with a slightly widened base and advances with slow, small steps. This is said to occur with Alzheimer's disease, multiple lacunar strokes (vascular dementia) and, occasionally, hydrocephalus. As dementia progresses the gait becomes stooped and shuffling and the associated arm-swinging is lost, the hands are held cupped, with the thumb adducted. Terminally, the patient cannot move his legs, is bedridden and assumes a flexed or cradled posture – 'paraplegia in flexion' – with hips and knees flexed toward the abdomen and the heels resting on the posterior thighs. Gait apraxia is a common presentation of normal pressure hydrocephalus.

Early dementia

The dementia syndrome, as we have seen stated repeatedly, is a constellation of clinical features. No one element, however distinctive in presentation, is indicative of dementia. If a patient presents with a history of failing memory, which is generally acknowledged to be an early feature – even though noted in retrospect usually – of dementia, the cause could be one of many, from being within limits of physiological normality to functional psychiatric disease. Even the advent of intellectual deterioration *or* a change of personality does not turn the presenting condition into dementia; one has to await the full panoply of symptoms. By the time all the features are assembled the dementing process might be anything but early, and one is often reduced to calling it 'mild'. Now, 'mild dementia' can apply to the early stages of the clinical syndrome but it throws little light on the underlying pathological process. We are almost completely unaware of what goes on between the onset of pathology and the full public display, as it were, of the clinical syndrome.

Bergmann (1979), referring to a study of an elderly group of patients in Newcastle, takes up some aspects of this difficulty. A group with 'suspected' dementia, with early or mild organic states, so designated because of their low score on memory and information tests, but nevertheless coping with their environment were followed up for an average of three years: 32% developed dementia, 37% turned out to be psychiatrically normal subjects of low IQ and social class leading a marginal and deprived existence, the remainder continued to be mildly impaired and of uncertain diagnostic status. In fact the largest number of subjects developing dementia came not from this group but from previously 'normal' and 'functional' groups in whom dementia had not been suspected. As Bergmann (1979) puts it:

> It seems likely therefore that not all elderly people with some degree of cognitive impairment will progress to frank dementia and that we shall have to distinguish between the clinical picture of early senile dementia of the Alzheimer type and other benign or less progressive forms of cognitive impairment.

In fact the World Health Organization Scientific Group on Psychogeriatric Classification (1972) suggested three sub-classifications under 'Atrophic senile psychoses': mild psycho-organic syndrome, moderate senile dementia

28

and severe senile dementia. This seems to beg the question somewhat but has the merit that a distinction is being made between dementia and other organic syndromes and the dementias in turn are classified descriptively according to severity, which is all that can be done with honesty in the present state of knowledge.

The early diagnosis of dementia has become a matter of some urgency for a number of reasons. Since it is rare for cases to present until the process has been going on for a period of some years we know far too little about its early manifestations, and yet logic dictates that for an attack on causation to be effective it has to be carried out in the case diagnosed early. Recent developments, which have opened up the possibility of chemical treatment for some forms and some symptoms of dementia, have added a special urgency to the need for intervention before the pathological process is advanced.

Another of the difficulties in establishing the early stages of dementia is posed by depression. The whole contentious issue of 'pseudo-dementia', especially that due to depressive illness, is dealt with at some length in Chapter 3. For the present the point may be made that depression may be a relatively common association with dementia as a symptom as well as being a harbinger of dementia. Its presence or exclusion may say nothing about a further, more organic, underlying pathology.

In the section on general clinical features, several symptoms, claimed as allegedly early features by some authors, were noted. The points made regarding depression are as applicable to these symptoms and the difficulties in assessing them are of a similar order.

Ultimately the problem of the early diagnosis of dementia is a conceptual one. By diagnosing a clinical condition and making it fit a conceptual framework we have constructed ourselves, all we can do as regards basic pathology is try to make an educated guess. Yet, as long as one goes on speaking about dementia, one has no alternative but to wait for the fully defined clinical picture to emerge, however promising any other result of investigations might be.

A way out of this dilemma might be to try to re-formulate the problem as a search for early diagnosis of pathology leading to dementia. This might involve psychometric assessment of what the psychologist defines as 'brain damage' and follow-up to find the patients who have turned out to be demented; computerized tomographic assessment of absorption density may have value as a predictor of dementia; electroencephalographic evidence of early slowing of the alpha rhythm, perhaps. None of these is a measure of early dementia, of course, but these or analogous parameters may reflect pathology that, in a proportion of cases, leads to the emergence of the full dementia syndrome. Retrospective examination of the data may then reveal those features, clinical as well as investigatory, that seemed to be present in the pre-demented state. The problems associated with some of these laboratory investigations are taken up in the respective chapters.

The last word on this subject must lie with neuropathological assessment. The best correlation between the clinical syndrome of dementia and any laboratory investigation is found with histopathological examination in

Alzheimer's disease. The correlation, though not perfect, is sufficiently close for the diagnosis of the disease to be made with reasonable conviction. Put in another way, follow-up of histologically determined Alzheimer's disease or a prodromal state, even in the asymptomatic or pre-demented state, may come close to the early stages of dementia we have been looking for. Our preoccupation with histopathology is, of course, for the present. Advances in histochemistry may provide us with a weapon of prospective value in attacking cases with early pathology who might not yield the full clinical picture of dementia until months or years later.

The difficulties with this line of attack are technical and ethical; in fact the two problems are related. But it is not all despair for a major advance in the technique of cerebral biopsy examination may remove ethical objections to the procedure in the same way the advent of computerized tomography has silenced the critics of pneumencephalography.

Senile dementia

In the present state of our knowledge – or ignorance as some might have it – 'senile dementia' can only be a descriptive term. One diagnoses dementia and then looks up the patient's date of birth. If he or she is 65 or over, the condition is senile dementia, if before, 'pre-senile'. The magic figure of 65 owes its existence to Otto Von Bismarck, the Chancellor of Germany, who in 1884 decreed it was the age at which citizens became entitled to their state old age pensions; the figure has been copied the world over and has enormous social and political significance. There is no discernible medical significance in this age.

As for the subtly different matter of a distinction in the nature of Alzheimer's disease presenting in the 'older' and the 'younger' patient, it remains a contentious business still, and is discussed in Chapter 3.

Course and outcome

Roth (1955) and Kidd (1962) found that elderly patients with senile psychosis, arteriosclerotic psychosis and acute confusion – all resulting from disease of the brain – had a two to three times higher mortality rate during the first 2 years of admission to hospital than those having such functional psychiatric disorders as affective psychosis or late paraphrenia.

Wang (1978) discusses the longevity in a group of patients with various brain diseases, summarized in Table 2.2.

Libow (1978) has provided a discussion on possible causes of death in Alzheimer's disease. They include (a) pneumonia (and other infections) – though he feels their incidence might have been exaggerated in some studies; (b) neglect by physicians and nurses ('benign neglect') – i.e. by discontinuing life-sustaining management and ordering a 'not to resuscitate' policy; (c) family collusion in the above; (d) misdiagnosis of associated illnesses; (e) an excessive use of medication; (f) malnutrition and dehydration; (g) a possible direct effect of dementia on other organs and (h) the somewhat, on present evidence, quaint notion that patients realize their hopeless state and go into terminal decline leading to death.

Table 2.2 Longevity in brain disease (after Wang, 1978, from several sources)

	Mean age at onset (years)	Mean age at death (years)	Observed survival (years)	Expected survival (years)
Senile dementia	71.3	77.3	6.0	11.1
Pre-senile dementia	53.8	60.7	6.9	22.3
Arteriosclerotic brain disease	66.8	71.4	3.8	13.4

Studies on the institutionalized elderly have related mortality to the number of errors in mental state examination, poor performance on tests of memory, decline in intelligence test scores and EEG abnormalities (Kaszniak *et al.*, 1978). Thus measures indicative of brain dysfunction are related to an increased death rate. However, most studies have not separated patients on the basis of diagnosis.

Kaszniak *et al.* (1978) studied 47 patients with a diagnosis of pre-senile or senile dementia and without focal neurological disease or major systemic illness who underwent a comprehensive assessment. They found that the degree of functional brain impairment, as detected on EEG – severe diffuse slowing and left temporal slowing – and neuropsychological assessment of memory and language function, rather than degree of cerebral atrophy, may be the more important influence on mortality in dementia patients without focal lesions. Also, short-term survival can be accurately predicted by tests of cognitive function, and expressive language deficit in such patients indicates a particularly poor prognosis for survival.

THE ASSESSMENT OF THE PATIENT WITH SUSPECTED DEMENTIA

A detailed format for the clinical assessment of the patient is given in the Appendix. Details for the investigation of the patient by psychometry, EEG, cerebral blood flow and computerized tomography will be found in the respective chapters on those topics. A few points, however, may be usefully made in concluding this chapter.

It will be clear from the preceding discussion that establishing a diagnosis of dementia is only the first step in the assessment of a patient with cognitive dysfunction. Further steps are required to

(1) discover or exclude a treatable cause of the dementia;

(2) ascertain any associated condition which might be aggravating the clinical picture or causing distress to the patient;

(3) enable the clinician to plan the wider management of a condition which, even when it is chronic and progressive, is not always of short duration and has serious implications for the family of the patient, the institutions of which he might become an inmate and for a wide range of social services if he continues to live in the community;

(4) assist studies on the various aspects of the syndrome that need to be

undertaken. It must be clear that the scope for research on dementia – reflecting, in effect, on our ignorance – must be vast and cannot be left to specialized centres alone. A careful, systematic, objective documentation of any aspect of dementia, in however simple or humble a form, must have its use. As with all other medical conditions, progress is likely only with attention being paid to fact and not by uninformed speculation or the pursuit of doctrine.

History

The onset and progress of both the syndrome of dementia and any suspected underlying cause of the condition must be established. It need hardly be said that while a history must be taken from the patient – in fact, it is part of the examination of the mental state – it will be grossly incomplete without a report from a reliable informant. An invariable feature of dementia is the partial or total loss of insight, poor memory, loss of intellect and change of personality, and a patient is usually unlikely to have the ability to fill in the picture by himself.

In the history it is important to note which of the symptoms of dementia emerged first and which later, and how they each progressed. A sceptical attitude is essential. One is dealing with matters which are hardly quantifiable in any objective fashion, even less by laymen, and repeated queries must be made as to whether the symptoms constitute a change from a previous state of normal well-being *for the patient*. A question on memory difficulty, for example, might elicit the answer 'he's always had a poor memory', which is more likely to have been a feature of premorbid personality rather than of present pathology.

As will be seen in the Appendix, the history of the present illness must be taken in addition to family history, past personal history, occupational and marital history, and past and present medical history, including intake of drugs and alcohol. The history concludes with an assessment of the premorbid personality which is possible only with reports from informants.

Examination

This is both physical and of the mental state.

Whilst the value of the history is not disputed, and is the single most important element in the assessment of the patient, the status of the neurological examination, around which so much mystique has grown, is more open to question. Fisher and Gonda (1955, quoted by Wells, 1980) reported that the neurological examination in 118 patients was falsely positive (meaning that it pointed out disease that could not be established) in 41% of cases and falsely negative (meaning that it failed to point to disease that was manifestly present) in 29%. Filskov and Goldstein (1974) have stated that the basic neurological examination was 'the least valid of all the physical procedures'. Caution is expressed in the evaluation of the following signs in the elderly: (a) small, poorly reactive pupils; (b) limited upward conjugate gaze; (c) muscular wasting, especially in the small muscles of the hands and feet; (d) intention or static tremor of the hands; (e) diminished appreciation of vibration distally in the lower extremities; (f) hypoactive muscle stretch reflexes (ankle jerks and superficial abdominal reflexes may even be absent); (g) akinetic, hypertonic changes with a general flexion attitude, poverty and slowness of movement (Wells, 1980).

Reviewing the evidence from which the foregoing and other findings emerged, Wells concludes that the value of the neurological examination as a diagnostic instrument is significantly limited by the frequency of both false-positives and false-negatives, perhaps more so in the elderly than in the younger age groups

Mental status examination

This refers to an examination of the patient's mental state at the time he is seen by the clinician. The patient must be seen alone, both to afford him the privacy to reveal what he can on even the most embarrassing of topics and also to prevent relatives rushing into answering the questions meant for the patient. It is implicit in the questions that the symptoms they refer to go back some time, usually a month or so: e.g. 'How have you been sleeping?' means over the past 4 weeks generally and not about any temporary difficulties of the previous day or two.

The importance of a general attitude of scepticism must be stressed; one starts off by assuming the patient is 'normal' and any evidence to the contrary must be adduced from the history and examination. When one is in doubt one must question the patient further and not be influenced by chance remarks and throwaway mutterings. One must also remember not to distress and fatigue the patient by questioning for too long. It is usually recommended that the average patient is not subjected to questioning beyond 50 minutes at any one session, and the elderly patient's limit is probably closer to half an hour. It follows from this that a swift diagnosis is not possible. The single biggest source of errors is probably the pressure to make a dash for diagnostic cover. If the diagnosis of dementia has to be an out-patient one, then several sessions may be required, but when one remembers that even in the earliest case of dementia presenting for assessment the pathological process has most likely been going on for some time, a delay of a few weeks in forming a clearer picture and a firm diagnosis is perfectly acceptable. Above all, the premorbid, or the usual, state of the patient, especially in terms of intellectual level, ability to remember and social behaviour, must be borne in mind. The clinician's interest is *change*, usually for the worst, in these parameters.

The psychiatric or mental state examination has been notoriously unreliable and for a long time was a constant source of irritation to those who wished to make sense of other people's findings, interpretations and conclusions. The opportunities for biased interviewing were unending and the reader is referred to Kendell (1975) for a flavour of the controversy.

For our purposes what is required is a validated set of questions in standardized form, with instructions for use, which can be used in several centres to obtain comparable results. Obviously its greatest value will be in research work, but there is an everyday need for simple, objective and reliable information. A very comprehensive semi-structured clinical interview for the assessment of the mental state in the elderly is available (Copeland *et al.*, 1976). It is called the Geriatric Mental State Schedule (GMSS) and is derived mainly from the Present State Examination (PSE) used on younger patients. It is, for reasons mentioned, primarily a research tool but there is no reason why the format and wording of the questions should not be studied with profit by anyone working with demented patients.

Investigations

Details of the commoner investigations undertaken on demented patients are given in chapters that follow, but a most revealing table from Wells (1980) might help put the whole subject in perspective (Table 2.3).

Table 2.3 Estimated efficiency of diagnostic techniques in identifying organic brain disease. (Scale 1–4; modified from Wells, 1980;) 1: most efficient; 4: least efficient.

Examination	False-positives	False-negatives
Neurological examination	2	3
Skull X-rays	1	4
EEG	1	3
CT	3	3
Psychological testing	3	1
CSF studies	1	4

Formulation

A patient with dementia or, for that matter, any condition, is not brought to a doctor simply for a laying on of diagnosis. Whilst a diagnosis is a satisfying intellectual exercise and possibly helps advance knowledge, it is only of indirect benefit to the patient. What he requires is for his difficulties to be understood and explained, and for steps to be taken to alleviate them. A formulation helps the doctor to do this. There is much talk of an arcane nature in psychiatric circles about the nature and function of the formulation. At its simplest the formulation is an attempt by the doctor to make sense of an individual patient by using all relevant information to hand. A practical method of doing this is discussed by Roth (1982). He lists his formulation under the headings of (1) primary diagnosis; (2) secondary descriptive diagnosis – any associated syndrome such as a depressive, manic or paranoid state or a secondary transient delirium; (3) aetiological diagnosis – e.g. cardiovascular, respiratory, etc., whether or not any causal relationship to dementia exists; (4) personality diagnosis – assessment of the patient's premorbid personality; (5) psychometric status – including both measurement of deficit as well as information useful in planning management; (6) assets and skills – social, domestic, personal and related to sphincters; (7) stance, gait and balance; (8) familial and social relationships and contacts.

It will be seen that the formulation enables one to deal with the whole individual who happens to suffer from dementia, and sets out the basis upon which rational management might be planned.

SUMMARY

(1) Dementia is due to an acquired, global impairment of intellect, memory and personality, in the absence of clouding of consciousness which leads to disorganization of several aspects of behaviour. Though commonly progressive and irreversible it is not necessarily so.

(2) The diagnosis, in the present conception of dementia, can only be made with regard to clinical criteria.

(3) As such, the use of laboratory criteria to make a diagnosis of dementia is untenable.

(4) If, however, the concept changes in the future, as it has often done in the past to take account of advancing knowledge, we may have to change our definition.

(5) Dementia, being a global condition present in the absence of clouding of consciousness, has to be distinguished from focal or localized disturbance of higher function (aphasia, dysmnesia) and cognitive impairment found in the presence of clouded consciousness (delirium).

(6) In terms of our present conception, early dementia must refer to the earliest stage at which the changes in cognition and behaviour satisfy the criteria for diagnosis of dementia. There need be no relation between the earliest detectable stage of dementia and the underlying pathology, which may be well advanced.

(7) Prognosis in most demented states is poor and the expected period of survival is considerably shortened. However, the growing number of treatable dementias is a source of encouragement.

(8) In the assessment of the patient suspected of having dementia the history, being an account of the onset and course of the illness, is crucial. As cognition is invariably involved, the information in the history must always be corroborated by independent witnesses.

(9) Laboratory investigations are important in the detection of the cause of dementia; in evaluating severity; in planning the management of the patient. False-positive and false-negative results are a constant source of difficulty.

(10) A formulation goes beyond the diagnosis, is an inventory of the patient's deficits and strengths and is the starting point for the rational planning of management.

Further reading

(A full list of references is given at the end of the book)

Lishman, W.A. (1978). *Organic Psychiatry*. (Oxford: Blackwell Scientific Publications)

Report of the Royal College of Physicians by the College Committee on Geriatrics (1981). Organic mental impairment in the elderly. *J. Roy. Coll. Phys. Lond.*, **15** (3), 141-167

Ropper, A.H. (1979). A rational approach to dementia. *Can. Med. Assoc. J.*, **121**, 1175-1190

Roth, M. (1980). Senile dementia and its borderlands. In Cole, J.O. and Barrett, J.E.(eds). *Psychopathology in the Aged*. (New York: Raven Press)

Roth, M. (1982). Perspectives in the diagnosis of senile and pre-senile dementia of Alzheimer type. In Sarner, M. (ed.) *Advanced Medicine*, **18**. (London: Pitman Medical)

3
The clinical features of the dementias

We are not ourselves
When nature, being oppress'd, commands the mind
To suffer with the body.

William Shakespeare (1564–1616),
King Lear, II, iv, 107-110

It is not possible at this stage in the study of dementia to provide a full aetiological classification of conditions giving rise to the syndrome. We have to be content with descriptive or aetiological criteria, or a combination of the two.

The Ninth Revision of the International Classification of Diseases (1978) classifies dementia under 'senile and pre-senile organic conditions' and 'other organic psychotic conditions (chronic)'. The former (290) includes senile dementia of the simple type, pre-senile dementia (including Alzheimer's disease and Pick's disease), senile dementia of the depressed or paranoid type, senile dementia with superimposed reversible episode of acute confusional state and arteriosclerotic dementia. 'Other organic psychotic conditions (chronic)' includes 'dementias in conditions classified elsewhere' which in turn takes in such conditions as Huntington's chorea and general paresis. It is advised that an additional code be used to certify the physical condition responsible.

One other point that needs to be made in this preamble is that disorders such as Alzheimer's disease which appear to be superficially homogeneous at present may well turn out to be a collection of disease processes with a common end point in discernible pathology and manifest symptomatology of dementia. To take Alzheimer's disease as an example again, though the condition commonly presents with a memory disturbance, other cases with prominent neurological features (bilateral pyramidal signs, release phenomena) and some with a parietal lobe syndrome have also been noted. So-called 'atypical' presentations are seen with other causes of dementia as well. This may suggest heterogeneity but at present we are not at all well placed, in most instances, to be certain.

37

It would seem sensible therefore to give a description of the clinical features of dementia in the following eclectic fashion.

To recapitulate the point made in the previous chapter, in assessing the patient the clinician establishes the presence of dementia by clinical and psychometric means and then pursues the causes of the dementia by recourse to the rest of the clinical picture and the results of investigations detailed in the following chapters.

Alzheimer's disease

This condition is probably the commonest cause of dementia; 50–60% of all cases of dementia, whether in the pre-senile or senile age groups, are thought to be due to Alzheimer's disease. Throughout this book, Alzheimer's disease has been used to describe the diagnosis made on histopathological grounds. 'Senile' and 'pre-senile' dementia have been terms employed to refer to any dementia that might occur in those above or below the age of 65, which might well be an arbitrary distinction. However, the features of Alzheimer's disease in the younger patient may differ from that in the aged and the evidence for this we shall examine later in this section.

Alzheimer's disease, though first described in a 51-year-old woman and believed to be the commonest of the pre-senile dementias, is now thought to occur at all ages. Since it is now clear that the propensity to dementia increases in general with age, especially in the period between 65 and 90 years, it is reasonable to assume that, contrary to previous belief, the older age groups show a higher incidence and prevalence of the condition though once again the caveat, that what we now know to be Alzheimer's disease might turn out to be a heterogeneous bag of conditions, must be entered into.

There is a female preponderance among both older and younger cases up to a ratio of 3 to 1 over males.

Most cases of Alzheimer's disease are sporadic but occasional clusters of familial cases, often with a pre-senile onset of the condition, have been reported. The case has been made over the years for dominant, recessive and multifactorial modes of transmission. The dominant mode of transmission has been noted especially in those families in which a significant number of members are afflicted. They are younger than the average case of Alzheimer's disease, males and females seem equally prone to be affected and a few distinctive neurological features restricted to the family involved may be seen.

Even though the majority of cases are sporadic there is clearly increased risk among first-degree relatives of patients, up to a factor of four. The alleged genetic distinction between Alzheimer's disease and senile dementia claimed by Larsson et al., (1963), after studying 2000 first-degree relatives of senile dementia and finding no case of Alzheimer's disease, has not been sustained by later work. Larsson et al. postulated an autosomal dominant transmission with limited penetrance.

The situation remains unclear but a growing consensus now favours a multifactorial mode of inheritance of the responsible genes, especially in sporadic cases. As so often with other conditions of polygenic inheritance, it could be that the greater the genetic loading, the earlier the onset of a sporadic illness and the more severe its subsequent course. This hypothesis would also allow a role for various environmental agents which are discussed in Chapter 8 in relation to the aetiological and pathogenetic influences they might have on Alzheimer's disease.

The clinical features of Alzheimer's disease are still best considered according to the plan laid out by Sjogren *et al.* (1952), who distinguished three stages in the development of the illness.

In the first stage, which may last 2–4 years, there is memory disturbance, spatial disorientation and a lack of spontaneity. The onset is usually insidious and it is rare for a patient to present with concern for the symptoms themselves. Social competence is preserved at this stage and the patient (and sometimes the relatives) often shows considerable resource-fulness in adapting to his difficulties or by making allowances. It is at this stage of the illness that depression and other changes of affect are most prominent, though this may soon proceed to apathy.

In the second stage there is a progressive involvement of the parietal lobe with the appearance of agnosia, aphasia and apraxia. It is also at this stage that the other two hallmarks of dementia, intellectual deterioration and personality change, become prominent. Neurological manifestations in the form of muscular weakness, extensor plantar response, disturbance of posture and gait with increased muscle tone and other features of parkinsonism may also be noted. If psychotic features such as delusions and hallucinations are seen, they too tend to make their appearance during this stage of the illness.

The third and terminal stage of the illness produces more severe neurological features. There is marked rigidity or spasticity. The reflexes may be released. Both grand mal seizures and myoclonic fits may be noted. By this time the patient is dulled into profound apathy, is doubly incontinent and wastes away.

The entire course of the average case of Alzheimer's disease lasts between 2 and 5 years. It is progressive and unremitting and there is no established treatment for any aspect of the condition. Clinical and psychometric observations often reveal an accentuation in the progression of the dementia in the few weeks before death.

For a diagnosis of Alzheimer's disease of the senile or pre-senile type, Roth (1982) believes three of the following four criteria must be satisfied:

(1) A gradual and progressive failure in the performance of work and in the common activities of life, which is not attributable to other disease conditions.

(2) Impairment in memory with difficulty in recording and retrieving recent personal experience and current information.

(3) Deterioration in general intellectual ability with impairment of grasp, capacity for reasoning, inference and abstract thought.

(4) Disorganization of personality with deterioration in self-care, emotional blunting, disinhibition and a coarsening of behaviour.

39

The exclusion criteria to be satisfied would be the elimination of other causes of dementia such as cerebrovascular disease, cerebral lesions due to specific causes or systemic diseases, deficiencies and intoxications liable to interfere with cerebral functioning (Roth, 1982). It will be appreciated that any attempt to make a diagnosis of Alzheimer's disease on this basis will simply be an educated guess. In the present state of knowledge the definitive diagnosis of the condition is by histopathology only.

Roth has also referred to the difficulties of making a diagnosis in early cases of dementia, where apathy, loss of initiative and a decline in general performance may lead to confusion with depression. Depressive symptoms in Alzheimer's disease are said to be of an isolated or fragmentary kind and confined to the early stages, after which they become even more tenuous and disappear. The subject of dementia due to depression ('pseudo-dementia') is taken up shortly.

It has already been suggested that differences might exist between Alzheimer's disease in older and younger patients. One of the differences claimed is that Alzheimer's disease in the younger or pre-senile patient might be a more severe affliction. Sourander and Sjogren (1970) showed that reduction in brain weight and neurofibrillary tangle presence were more severe in pre-senile Alzheimer patients than in senile dementia, with better-preserved physical bodily status in the younger patient.

The other distinctive feature claimed is the presence of focal parietal lobe dysfunction manifested in such symptoms as aphasia, apraxia, agnosia and acalculia in the younger patient. These tend to come on in the first couple of years of the condition when memory deficit and failing performance of everyday tasks are already present.

There is also a suggestion that the temporal lobe might be implicated, especially in the younger patient. Sourander and Sjogren (1970) have drawn attention to the presence of a phenomenon in Alzheimer's disease which corresponds to the Kluver Bucy syndrome following bilateral temporal lobe excision in monkeys. The features include visual agnosia with an inability to recognize faces of self and others, the tendency to mouth objects (hyperorality) and to touch every object in sight (hypermetamorphosis). Indiscriminate eating (hyperphagia) and an emotional apathy and blunting corresponding to the tameness of the monkeys with the syndrome are other features. The authors believe that in most cases (up to 75%) these features form part of the essential symptomatology of Alzheimer's disease, though they may also be seen in Pick's disease and cerebral tumours.

Another feature often commented on in pre-senile cases is the incidence of florid neurological phenomena such as upper and lower motor neurone signs, parkinsonism and both grand mal and myoclonic seizures. Sir Martin Roth has observed that quite apart from being a possible point of distinction between two age-related forms of Alzheimer's disease this observation may heighten interest in a study of any link between Alzheimer's disease and the transmissible dementias. It must be stressed that at present there is no evidence that Alzheimer's disease is transmissible.

Taking all these factors into consideration, it may be permissible to postulate that there are two forms, if not types, of Alzheimer's disease. It has been argued that age might be the crucial factor, with early-onset and late-onset forms of the disease. but age could be just one variable, with the severe form having an onset earlier in patients at greater genetic risk. Quite apart from age and other clinical features, forms of Alzheimer's disease running a severe and less severe course – it is hardly possible to suggest that any form of Alzheimer's disease runs a benign course – seem distinct on a variety of investigations. The degree of radiodensity attenuation in the right parietal region on CT scanning corresponds to clinical scores of dysphasia, dysgraphia and dyspraxia and predicts those patients who died among a group of senile dements on follow-up (Naguib and Levy, 1982).

Similarly, expressive language deficit indicates a particularly poor prognosis for survival (Kaszniak *et al.*, 1978). This series also showed that left-sided temporal slowing on the EEG was predictive of death within a year. It has also been shown (Bird *et al.*, 1983) that myoclonus, while being a feature of younger patients with more severe Alzheimer's disease, was also the single best predictor of low brain choline acetyl transferase.

If the presence of focal and cortical symptomatology is a major and early feature of the severe form of Alzheimer's disease, is the difference between the two forms that between cortical and subcortical dementia? The essential clinical difference between 'subcortical' dementia – a concept put forward to take account of the features of cognitive dysfunction and personality change in such conditions as progressive supra-nuclear palsy, Parkinson's disease and Huntington's chorea (and discussed later in this chapter) – and 'cortical' dementia of the more usual kind is the lack of features of dysphasia, dyspraxia and dysgnosia in the former. A recent study (Mayeux *et al.*, 1983) in which Alzheimer's disease was diagnosed clinically – i.e. with the exclusion of focal, and hence the more severe, features – showed that there was no distinctive pattern of neuropsychological impairment between Alzheimer's disease, Huntington's chorea and Parkinson's disease.

It may also be proposed that there is a reciprocal relationship between the nature and intensity of depressive symptoms and the course and prognosis of an associated dementing illness. When the depression is prominent, well-differentiated and responsive to treatment the dementia has a relatively better prognosis; when it is fleeting, poorly differentiated and unresponsive to treatment, the prognosis of the dementia is particularly poor. It is interesting in this context that Geriatric Mental State Schedule scores for 'somatic concern' and 'obsessional symptoms' – suspected by the authors of reflecting depression – were higher in a group of survivors than in a comparable group of dements who died (Naguib and Levy, 1982). Also, when dements and depressives share an abnormality in the dexamethasone suppression test, it would appear it is the slower-progressing cases of Alzheimer's disease that are related in this respect to depressive illness (Mahendra, 1984). The extent of histopathological and neurochemical differences between the two forms of Alzheimer's disease is discussed in Chapter 8.

Alzheimer's disease was first described and studied as the commonest variety of pre-senile dementia and interest persists in attempting to distinguish it from other pre-senile causes of dementia in anticipation of histopathology. In Alzheimer's disease memory difficulties present early and almost invariably precede other changes. Other common manifestations are the emotional changes which progress from depression or anxiety to apathy and spontaneity. Another characteristic feature, though commoner in the younger patient, is parietal lobe dysfunction in the form of apraxia, aphasia and agnosia. Sim *et al.* (1966) have noted those features which occur early in other pre-senile dementias and might help distinguish them from Alzheimer's disease, where they occur late, rarely or not at all. These include fits, incontinence, confabulation, personality change, delusions and hallucinations and gross focal neurological disturbance such as spasticity, hemiparesis, striatal rigidity and tremor.

The distinction between Alzheimer's disease and Pick's disease might also be made with the help of Table 3.1.

The value of laboratory and other investigatory techniques in helping to make this distinction is discussed in the following chapters.

Table 3.1 Distinguishing features between Alzheimer's disease and Pick's disease (After Glen and Christie, from Robertson, 1978)

Alzheimer's disease	Pick's disease
1. Predilection for parietal and hippocampal area involvement proceeding to global brain atrophy.	1. Atrophy predominates in frontal and temporal areas.
2. Onset primarily with memory deficit.	2. Onset primarily with personality change with preservation of topographical memory. Euphoria frequent.
3. Progression to loss of topographical sense and dyspraxia.	3. Topographical sense preserved till late. Dyspraxia minimal or absent.
4. Psychotic manifestations and seizures not uncommon.	4. Psychotic episodes and seizures seldom found.
5. Hyperalgesia uncommon.	5. Hyperalgesia often present.

VASCULAR (ALSO ARTERIOSCLEROTIC OR MULTI-INFARCT) DEMENTIA

The multiple titles are indicative of the nosological and aetiological confusion surrounding the subject. The older adjective 'arteriosclerotic' is a misnomer anyway, as pathology cannot be attributed to a physiological process. What was presumably meant was dementia due to atherosclerosis but the relationship between atheromatous changes in the larger arteries and dementia is far from clear. There is little evidence that stenosis or occlusion of the carotid arteries and a subsequent impairment in the blood supply by itself is instrumental in initiating a dementing process except by producing infarction and the necessary damage to brain structures that results in dementia.

Tomlinson *et al.* (1968) have shown that up to 40% of subjects over 65 years showing no evidence of intellectual deterioration prove at autopsy to have cerebral infarctions. The presence of stenosis or occlusion of the carotid arteries is also a not uncommon post-mortem finding but when demented and non-demented subjects are studied in relation to large vessel pathology there is no difference in the extent of the involvement of the vessels. It must, however, be pointed out, as was done by Harrison *et al.*(1979), that when a series of demented patients were divided into an 'ischaemic' group and a 'primary degenerative' group, there was angiographic evidence of ischaemic areas and atheromatous disease of intracranial vessels to a greater extent in the 'ischaemic' group.

'Multi-infarct' is a descriptive term but suffers from the slight disadvantage that it can only be applied to a diagnosis of dementia following autopsy or computerized tomography. Moreover, multiple infarcts may be found without dementia (in strokes, for example) and dementia, even in the presence of all other presumed features of vascular origin, can exist without visible infarction.

To add a further twist to this confused and disputatious terminology, it has now been suggested (see Chapter 8) that dementia might be due to disturbed homeostasis, which, it is claimed, is usually mediated through changes in capillary permeability. Clearly, 'vascular' dementia may have yet another dimension.

Inevitably there has been an overdiagnosis of the prevalence of vascular dementia. Corsellis (1969) has pointed out that in the middle-aged adult the clinical diagnosis of vascular dementia is encountered much more often than is justified by the eventual pathological findings. In the aged patient it seems the relatively common minor infarctions described earlier will produce the clinical evidence of focal disorder which leads to an erroneous diagnosis of vascular dementia.

It is not difficult to understand the reasons for this over-diagnosis. The traditional method of distinguishing vascular dementia from non-vascular dementia is by applying a set of clinical rules, nowadays put into the rather formal Hachinski's Ischaemic Score (see below). Any demented patient who scores 7 and over is designated 'vascular'. These rules must in the nature of things lead to an increase in the diagnosis of vascular dementia though Roth (1982) believes that recent studies of the neuropathology of the brain at post-mortem examination have on the whole validated the effectiveness of these criteria.

Several causes of vascular dementia have been enumerated. Some are relatively common, some rare and a few have yet to be established beyond dispute. Caplan (1979) has said that, in addition to disease of the larger cerebral vessels, hypertensive disease of the small vessels may result in vascular dementia. In some cases, he has said, widespread cerebral infarction may result from inadequate cerebral perfusion in the absence of serious intrinsic disease of the cerebral vessels. Other alleged causes include clotting disorders and vasculitis, multiple cerebral embolization even if only occult in nature, cardiac causes such as recent myocardial infarctions, rheumatic mitral sterosis with atrial fibrillation, bacterial endocarditis, marantic endocarditis, myocardiopathy with mural thrombosis, ventricular aneurysms and atrial fibrillation with recurrent embolization (Caplan, 1979).

Hachinski *et al.* (1974) have referred to certain uncommon conditions which may produce vascular dementia through the common denominator of multiple cerebral infarcts. These include collagen vascular disease, Takayasu disease, moya-moya disease and progressive small-vessel occlusions described by Torvik. Scheinberg (1978) has added fibromuscular dysplasia with bilateral carotid artery thombosis.

The vascular dementias are found in both males and females but with a slight male preponderance, unlike Alzheimer's disease which occurs considerably more commonly in females. There is no clear genetic relationship discernible except secondarily through hypertension and atheromatous disease, which is commoner in men. It begins in late middle age and in the senium though cases may be seen in the forties and fifties.

The onset is usally sudden and a common presentation is after a cerebrovascular accident, when the additional disability draws attention to gradual changes which might have been concealed by the patient or been played down by relatives. Some of those slower-evolving changes might have involved affective symptoms. These may precede cognitive symptoms and include, apart from depression and anxiety, lability and explosive and short-lived emotional outbursts. Emotional lability is often described as a characteristic feature and is attributed to involvement of the basal regions of the brain. The patient laughs and weeps upon minor provocation.

Somatic symptoms, including headache and dizziness, may amount to what is thought to be a picture of hypochondriasis and are also believed to be a distinctive feature of this form of dementia.

Cognitive changes, as has been suggested, are less prominent than in Alzheimer's disease and run a fluctuating course. A typical feature, often described and whose significance is still not clear, is nocturnal confusion and agitation. The psychological deficits which result in between exacerbations of mental state are patchy. The personality is relatively well preserved as is a surprising degree of insight. This is, of course, a mixed blessing for the patient, and the emotional changes including the severe depression that has been noted in the condition have been attributed to patients being aware of their condition.

A cardinal feature of the condition is the presence of focal neurological features. These appear episodically and their sequela is a progressively worsening dementia. Florid neurological signs such as aphasia or hemiparesis may be present. In their absence, Birkett (1972) has described the presence of minor focal signs such as unequal tendon reflexes, extensor plantar responses or impaired pupil reactions. Parkinsonian features, pseudo-bulbar palsy and epileptic seizures may also be found.

A characteristic feature of the commoner variety of vascular dementia is the course it follows. Unlike Alzheimer's disease which results in progressive deterioration, in vascular dementia there is described a 'step-wise' progression of the condition. Episodic exacerbations are followed by a plateau, even by mild remission, soon to be followed by another exacerbation. Remissions soon cease and the patient, in between attacks, continues to function at a very low level of performance.

The period of survival is generally longer than in Alzheimer's disease though occasionally a rapid course can be followed by sudden death. Roth (1955) showed that at 6 months following admission to an institution arteriosclerotic dementia patients seemed to be doing better than senile dementia patients, though at the end of 2 years there was little difference and more than two-thirds of the patients with arteriosclerotic dementia were dead. Females with arteriosclerotic dementia are thought to fare better than those with Alzheimer's disease.

Death occurs on the average after 5–6 years following diagnosis and is usually due to one of the manifestations of a generalized atheromatous process, ischaemic heart disease, cerebrovascular accident or renal disease.

Roth (1982) has paid special attention to the features in the clinical presentation of vascular dementia with special reference to diagnostic difficulty. Hachinski *et al.* (1975) had converted the main diagnostic features of vascular or multi-infarct or arteriosclerotic dementia as described by several writers, including Slater and Roth (1969), into an 'ischaemia score' which they used clinically on patients diagnosed as demented to differentiate 'primary degenerative dementia' from 'multi-infarct dementia'. The 'ischaemia score' is shown in Table 3.2.

Table 3.2   Ischaemia score (after Hachinski *et al.*, 1975)

Abrupt onset	2	Emotional lability	1
Stepwise deterioration	1	Hypertension	1
Fluctuation	2	History of stroke	2
Nocturnal confusion	1	Focal symptoms	2
Relative preservation of personality	1	Focal signs	2
Depression	1	Other signs of arteriosclerosis	1
Somatic complaints	1		

The 'cut-off' score is 7, and it is said that it is possible by this means to identify about 50% of ischaemic cases correctly. Roth (1982) believes a sharper discrimination and an improved diagnostic scale might have been possible with the aid of a discriminant function analysis and a differential weighting of the features of value. These include abrupt onset, fluctuating course, history of focal symptoms and focal signs, presence of depression, emotional lability and 'other signs of arteriosclerosis', all of which seem to distinguish multi-infarct or vascular dementia patients from Alzheimer's disease patients.

Roth has also said a criterion relating to duration of symptoms might be useful, as in vascular dementia the history of intellectual decline is shorter than in Alzheimer's disease. There is also a call to sharpen up the index for 'step-wise deterioration'. The first few strokes the patient suffers may leave him with transient cognitive impairment or none; it is only later that increasingly severe and enduring impairment of intellectual function occurs.

Taking up the other features, Roth has commented that 'fluctuation' refers to the periodic return to relatively efficient intellectual functioning and good or normal emotional rapport that characterizes the condition in the first few years when therapeutic intervention might still be possible; 'depression' in multi-infarct or vascular dementia may respond to treatment at least for limited periods, unlike that associated with senile dementia of the Alzheimer type; 'hypertension' has to be severe, systolic/diastolic of 200/100, to be of value in distinction; 'other signs of arteriosclerosis' may

include angina pectoris, previous myocardial infarction, intermittent claudi-
cation or retinal artery thrombosis. 'Focal symptoms and signs' are of
unequivocal diagnostic value.

The conventional distinction between Alzheimer's disease and vascular
dementia is made in Table 3.3. The features described already are those to
be found in the common variety of vascular dementia, known in the past as
'arteriosclerotic' dementia and more recently as 'multi-infarct' dementia.
Two variants of this state now need to be discussed.

Heyman (1978) and Caplan (1979) have described the 'lacunar state'
which consists of multiple cystic infarcts varying in size from 2 to 10 mm
and almost invariably related to hypertension and atherosclerosis. Some
lacunar infarcts produce clinical strokes, others are relatively silent. Fisher
(1965) has emphasized that the presence of such lesions need not necessarily
lead to mental deterioration. In his series of 1000 autopsies, multiple
lacunae were found in about 10% but only a fifth of those had shown any
neurological features, let along dementia, during life. However, it is believed
that multiple lacunae can gradually destroy the basal ganglia, thalamus and
the deep cerebral white matter, the results being additive in effect. The
clinical features include a past history compatible with small vessel disease,
i.e. hypertension and diabetes mellitus; a history of acute deficits in the form
of strokes; parkinsonism but without the tremor, bilateral pyramidal signs
and pseudobulbar palsy with emotional lability, dysarthria and dysphagia.
Computerized tomography reveals small lesions compatible with lacunae,
enlarged ventricles and white matter loss, occasionally in the presence of a
preserved cortical mantle.

When a more diffuse lesion involving gross scarring of white matter, basal
grey matter and severe small vessel disease occurs, a condition called
'subcortical arteriosclerotic encephalopathy' (Binswanger's disease) is
thought to exist. Binswanger (1894) described eight patients under what he
termed 'encephalitis subcorticalis chronica progressiva' due to an atherosclerotic deficiency in blood flow. Several authors in recent years (Caplan
and Schoene, 1978; Caplan, 1979; Loizou et al., 1981) have described the
clinical features of the condition. These include an association with
hypertension of a moderate or severe degree, a presentation with strokes but
also with a more subacute progression of a focal deficit over weeks or
months, epileptic fits, pseudobulbar palsy, hydrocephalus, long plateau
periods over which the deficit improves or remains stable, prominent motor
signs and a slowly developing dementia in patients in the 50–60 age group.
The pathology seems to affect predominantly the perforating vessels to the
subcortical grey and white matter with multiple areas of infarction and
diffuse myelination. There is relative sparing of the cortex. Loizou et al.
(1981) believe the white matter low attenuation with mild atrophy and
infarction may well be a significant feature on computerized tomography of
this condition and, along with the subacute accumulation of deficits,
provide points of distinction from the lacunar state with which it can be
readily confused. They also note that subacute deficits and white matter low
attenuation have not been noted in 'multi-infarct' dementia.

Although the stark descriptions in these sections might give the impression (potentiated by Table 3.3) that the clinical distinction between vascular dementia and Alzheimer's disease is readily made, this is, of course, not true in practice where considerable difficulties are often experienced. It is more than an academic problem, for it is reasonable to assume that a substantial proportion of vascular dementias are associated with, or causally related to, hypertension and multiple embolic phenomena, and may thus be susceptible to medical or surgical intervention, which is not the case with Alzheimer's disease.

Caplan (1979) has provided a simple basis for a rational understanding of the differences between these two major causes of dementia. There is early and prominent involvement of motor, visual and sensory pathways in the vascular dementias, Caplan believes, because vascular occlusion affects both the areas required for the survival of the organism (motor function, vision, hearing, etc.) and those regions subserving higher function. This is in contrast to senile dementia in which a presumably more selective process attacks speech, memory and visuospatial function well before motor, sensory, visual or reflex function. Acute strokes produce an abruptly developing deficit which then improves while the atrophy of Alzheimer's disease leads to a slowly progressive course. There is also the presence of asymmetric and 'patchy' dysfunction in vascular lesions with gross disability in one area of function and preservation in another. This is understandable in terms of the focal deficits which arise from the lesion.

The differences between vascular or multi-infarct dementia and Alzheimer's disease on investigation are taken up in the respective chapters.

Pick's disease

This was in fact the second of the great quartet of pre-senile dementias (the others being Huntington's chorea (1872), Alzheimer's disease (1907) and Creutzfeldt–Jakob disease (1920, 1921)) to be described in 1892, but when confusion arises it is usually with Alzheimer's disease which is a far commoner cause of pre-senile dementia.

Genetic transmission is thought to be through a single autosomal dominant gene and women are affected twice as often as men. As a pre-senile dementia it occurs between the ages of 50 and 60, though cases have been described in younger patients.

The clinical features tend to reflect the neuropathological findings reported in the condition and, in contrast to the memory difficulties found commonly in Alzheimer's disease, frontal lobe involvement is a common early feature in Pick's disease. This manifests itself in a change of personality and aberrant social behaviour. Drive is lost and tactless, insensitive and disinhibited behaviour may occur. Social and sexual disinhibition may lead to alcoholism as well as criminal activity. This grossly deteriorated behaviour includes a tendency to pranks and cruel or humourless jokes. There is an early loss of insight and the prevailing mood is often described as fatuous, though euphoria may be noted as well. Incontinence may occur early and is popularly attributed to frontal lobe involvement.

Impairment of memory and intellect is observed at a later stage than in

Table 3.3   The distinction between vascular dementia and Alzheimer's disease.

Vascular dementia	Alzheimer's disease
1. Found among 10–15% of representative cases of dementia.	1. Probably the commonest cause of presenile and senile dementia.
2. Males more commonly affected.	2. Females more commonly affected.
3. No clear genetic involvement.	3. Genetic contribution suspected.
4. Relatively sudden onset.	4. Insidious onset.
5. Step-wise progression.	5. Gradual and progressive course.
6. Somatic complaints common.	6. Somatic complaints, as opposed to physical disability, rare.
7. Evidence of focal neurological disease present.	7. Evidence of focal disease not usually present.
8. Hypertension and fits more common.	8. Hypertension and fits less common.
9. Evidence for generalized atheromatous disease often present.	9. Little evidence for generalized atheromatous disease.
10. Relatively good preservation of personality.	10. Personality disintegration a marked feature.
11. Insight relatively well preserved.	11. Insight lost early.
12. Marked affective change including depression, anxiety and lability.	12. Affect blunted after early stages.

Alzheimer's disease. A feature which has been commented upon is a relative sparing of constructional and visuospatial ability in the early stages, which also helps to distinguish it from Alzheimer's disease in which they are lost early.

There is an earlier speech involvement than with Alzheimer's disease and the left hemisphere generally may be incriminated to a greater extent than the right. There is marked perseveration of speech and stereotyped repetition of brief words and phrases is described as being characteristic, though they may alternate with mutism. Aphasia is less common and, as with other parietal lobe signs such as apraxia and agnosia, occurs less frequently than in Alzheimer's disease. Gait, tone and extrapyramidal disturbance generally are also less common. Delusions, hallucinations and epileptic fits are rare.

Computerized tomography may show a dissociated atrophy between the temporofrontal and other lobes and the EEG is said to be near normal in early cases.

Many of the points of distinction recorded above apply only to early cases as with the progress of the condition Pick's disease comes to resemble most other cases of dementia. The period of survival is longer than in Alzheimer's disease and may be up to 10 years though the average is closer to 5 years.

Some points in the clinical distinction between Alzheimer's disease and Pick's disease are tabulated (Table 3.1) and the features found on investigation are described in the respective chapters.

HUNTINGTON'S CHOREA

This disease, described officially in 1872 though observed for several years previously, has been reported from the world over and is notorious for the florid nature of both psychiatric and neurological manifestations as well as the dementia. Its prevalence is discussed in Chapter 10 and some aspects of the management of this condition are referred to in Chapter 9. More than with most other conditions, aspects of epidemiology and management complement clinical description.

The account in this section is based on the description given by the Office of Health Economics (1980).

Huntington's chorea occurs equally in both sexes and is thought due to a single autosomal dominant gene with virtually 100% manifestation in survivors. The risk to offspring is 50% at birth and this falls to a much lower figure by the age of 70 years (see Chapter 10). There is thought also to be an anticipation, with succeeding generations having a progressively earlier onset, via the paternal line. The evidence for this seems to be that child victims of the disease inherit a disproportionately large number of cases from their fathers and that, even amongst adults, in affected offspring of male Huntington's chorea victims death occurs at an earlier age than with offspring of female victims.

However, a family history may be apparently absent in up to 20% of cases. Mutations are often blamed but it is thought that less than 5% of cases can be attributed to this cause. It is more likely that denial of knowledge of the illness (both conscious and otherwise), illegitimacy (promiscuity and increased fertility are often seen as a result of the disease) and unaccounted-for deaths are more likely sources of an incomplete family history.

The age of onset of the condition is between 35 and 40 years though the range can be considerable; 2% of cases occur below 10 years of age and 10% in the seventh decade. Within a given family the age of onset, the symptoms and the rate of decline are in general consistent.

It is generally believed that behavioural changes appear first, then chorea, and the dementia follows these features. Once again, as with age of onset, it is stressed that wide variation is possible. In the earliest stage there may be significant changes in personality with irritability, querulousness, apathy and a disregard for other people being marked features. Paranoid personality change has been noted. Florid schizophreniform and depressive psychoses are one source of diagnostic error in the period preceding chorea and dementia. Paranoia manifesting itself as morbid jealousy is a source of danger to the spouse and domestic violence in the family of Huntington's chorea patients is a feature very familiar to those managing patients and their families. Depression is, however, the commoner psychiatric manifestation and suicide is a real prospect, as Huntington observed in his original remarks on the condition. Suicide is thought to account for 7% of deaths amongst Huntington's chorea patients and in the US the suicide rate among the families of patients is thought to be about seven times the national average. Other behavioural disorders that have been reported in Huntington's chorea patients and their families are self-mutilation, serious crime, alcoholism and sexual disturbance. Divorce and separation, promiscuity and illegitimacy may also be causes of difficulty in the family.

Chorea usually precedes dementia but the one very occasionally may be present without the other. Before the full-blown choreic picture is noted, clumsiness, fidgetiness and unsteadiness may be seen. The subject's attempts to disguise this may exacerbate the appearance of restlessness. The face is involved in the form of mannerisms and everyday activity becomes difficult. The movements then become abrupt and jerky and the facial expression can become grotesque on account of the contortions of the facial muscles. The fingers, arms and shoulders may also become affected and the gait disturbance is a prominent feature. When accompanied by slurred speech, alcoholic intoxication becomes the suspected diagnosis to the casual observer. As the illness advances the chorea increases in severity and virtually all muscles become involved. The movements seem worse on voluntary or deliberate activity and walking, eating and sitting become difficult.

Hemichorea may affect half the body and dysphagia, with the risk of choking, may occur with the spread of involuntary movement.

Occasionally, especially in the younger patient, extrapyramidal signs may develop in addition to the chorea, rarely in the absence of it, with akinesia, tremor and rigidity. Parkinson's disease is a mistaken diagnosis, as are multiple sclerosis, Wilson's disease, cerebellar lesions and drug toxicity.

Dementia follows the early psychiatric features and the chorea and is insidious in its development. A general inefficiency, often attributable to the psychiatric symptoms, is more in evidence than in Alzheimer-type memory disability. In fact there tends to be a relative preservation of the memory as opposed to personality and intellectual disorientation. Focal features such as dysphasia and dyspraxia are not shown though, surprisingly, dyscalculia is sometimes present. As will be discussed later, the dementia of Huntington's chorea conforms to what has been called 'subcortical' dementia. Insight, too, may be preserved to a later extent than in the equivalent case with Alzheimer's disease. The condition progresses to apathy and inertia which may, however, be punctuated with outbursts of violent excitement which may be difficult to manage.

The period of survival in Huntington's chorea depends on the age of onset of the condition. As we shall see shortly, childhood affliction leads to death on average within 6–7 years but in middle age the life expectancy is about 15 years on average. The variation, once again, is wide.

Variants of the classical picture are seen in childhood and in young adults. Though there is little doubt that Huntington's chorea can occur in childhood, there can be no dementia in the strict interpretation of the definition. The mental decline before the age of 16 must be considered a species of mental handicap.

Juvenile Huntington's chorea involves between 3% and 5% of cases, with perhaps 1% of all cases occurring below 10 years of age. The first signs are clumsiness and unsteadiness, which progress only rarely to chorea. Rigidity, tremor and hypokinesia are more frequent. There is rapid mental deterioration and epilepsy is a prominent feature in more than 50% of cases. The mean time of survival is halved and diagnostic errors (the condition being confused with Wilson's disease, Friedreich's ataxia, epilepsy and other causes of acquired mental deficit) are not uncommon. The infant and childhood mortality among unaffected children born into Huntington's chorea families is high. This may be due to unidentified disease but the seriously disorganized state of the family in this illness is also likely to play a part.

The second variant occurs in young adults and was first described by Westphal in 1905. Tremor is an early symptom, and progresses to violent trembling on voluntary movement. There is muscular rigidity and hypokinesia as well. A characteristic abnormality in some of these cases is said to be an inability to move the eyes, which leads to a fixed (old-fashioned) 'doll's eye' gaze.

CREUTZFELDT–JAKOB DISEASE (CJD)

Aspects of this very intriguing illness have been discussed in the chapters on history, pathology and epidemiology. Discovery of the illness and the first descriptions of it are usually traced to Creutzfeldt (1920) and Jakob (1921) but considerable doubt is now expressed as to whether they described cases which we would now call CJD.

CJD presents as a dementing illness running a rapid course after evolving over weeks and months, and is accompanied by pyramidal, extrapyramidal and cerebellar signs. Though most cases are thought to be sporadic in origin, up to 15% of all cases of CJD seem to have a family history of disease consistent with autosomal dominant transmission (Masters *et al.*, 1979). One instance of husband and wife being affected has also been reported. The evidence for a transmissible agent for the illness is now compelling.

Males and females are affected to the same extent. CJD may occur in the first and second decades but the commoner decade of onset is the fourth or fifth. It is earlier in familial cases. The prodromal symptoms are vaguely somatic with apathy, malaise, insomnia, depression and anxiety which may lead to a suspicion of functional psychiatric illness. The first firm evidence of CJD seems to come by way of sensomotor disintegration, i.e. disturbances of stance, gait and motor control, visual disturbances, dizziness and vertigo which precede the dementia. These early symptoms may remit and return.

There is great diversity in the neurological picture and tendency of the symptoms to change as the disease evolves adds to the confusion and diagnostic doubt. Neurological signs include cerebellar ataxia, spasticity, rigidity, inco-ordination, myoclonus, tremor, choreoathetosis, small muscle wasting and fibrillation, parietal lobe symptoms, cortical blindness, dysarthria, bulbar palsy and epileptic fits.

Memory difficulties and intellectual deterioration usually follow the neurological changes but evolve very rapidly and soon catch up with the physical changes. As the dementia progresses, myoclonus may emerge and the appearance of myoclonus in rapidly advancing dementia is particularly suggestive of CJD. Elation, hallucinations and delusions have been reported but are soon overtaken by a severe dementia which is accompanied by emaciation. The EEG (see Chapter 5) may become distinctive in about 70% of cases at a later stage in the illness with 'triphasic' bursts on a slow background.

51

The illness runs a very rapid course and most patients are dead within 2 years. The mean age of death is given as 57 years (Masters *et al.*, 1979).

It is usual to think of Kuru in the same breath as CJD but Kuru, despite an involvement of the cortex, differs from CJD in not producing a profound dementia. Its features are severe cerebellar ataxia and tremor. It is also customary to seek variants of cases of CJD, e.g. a syndrome with occipital cortical involvement and another with cerebellar signs. Masters and Gajdusek (1982) have disputed the validity of making these distinctions, claiming that an analysis of these types of cases shows an overlapping of clinical and pathological features to an extent that such subclassifications have little practical benefit.

However, some of these variants will be described briefly at a purely descriptive level. Jakob himself seems to have described one of these, a case with motor neurone disease, spasticity, dementia and extrapyramidal features. These syndromes of motor neurone disease with dementia, in the absence of typical spongiform encephalopathy, are grouped together under the heading of *amyotrophic CJD* (Masters and Gajdusek, 1982). Another variant described in the past is *subacute spongiform encephalopathy*, occurring in an older patient with degeneration of the visual striate cortex, severe myoclonic fits and a devastating course with a rapid, fatal termination. Another is the *cerebellar ataxic* variant, with rapidly progressive ataxia and myoclonus in addition to a severe dementia.

In a recently published retrospective study of 121 cases of Creutzfeldt–Jakob disease, Will and Matthews (1984) distinguished three varieties of presentation – by far the most common was the *subacute form*, rapidly leading to a helpless condition and early death. The onset was vague and non-specific, but the commonest symptom at presentation for medical advice was impairment of higher mental function or behavioural disturbance. Frank neurological symptoms and signs followed later. The characteristic course in these patients was of rapid deterioration to a decorticate state that might persist for several months before death. In the *intermediate* group the cases were of heterogeneous presentation with duration of illness ranging from 20 months to 16 years and with varying clinical features. In the *amyotrophic* form the course was more stereotyped, with slowly progressive dementia over a period of 1–7 years prior to the development of wasting and fasciculation of limbs or bulbar musculature. Deterioration was more rapid, resulting in death within a year, and myoclonus was not a feature in these patients.

'PSEUDO-DEMENTIA'

The assumption up to now in this study of dementia has been that even if the causes of the dementias were not always known, the presence of brain pathology was reasonably well described. However, the clinical syndrome of dementia also includes a variable number of cases which satisfy the requirements of the definition of dementia but have no discernible (by the application of techniques in the present state of knowledge, that is) 'organic' brain lesion. This group, which consists largely of patients with depressive illness but may include those with schizophrenia, mania, the neuroses and other psychiatric illness, comes under the conventional heading of 'functional' illness and the dementia they give rise to is usually known as 'pseudo-dementia', in contrast to the 'true dementia' of organic origin.

It is precarious terminology, for even the most casual reading of medical history must reveal the changing and improving methods of ascertaining brain pathology. We have seen investigation of the brain move from macroscopic dissection to light microscopy to ultrastructural histology and a histochemical assault on brain disease. What is not revealed today does not necessarily stay unrevealed tomorrow. In any case, several workers might dispute that even today all cases of depression and so-called functional psychiatric disease are truly 'functional' and point to the growing, if admittedly still incomplete, evidence of brain pathology in some of these conditions. For instance Kety (1967, 1972) has suggested that noradrenergic neurones may play a role in sustaining mood and mental activity, memory and learning and thus a dysfunction in that system could be common to both depression and dementia.

But in a study of dementia at present these considerations are almost irrelevant. It has been shown at some length in Chapter 2 that the present-day concept of dementia is a clinical one, descriptive but not aetiological. The clinician's first duty is to assess the mental changes in the patient and decide if a diagnosis of dementia can be upheld in terms of the defining criteria of the syndrome. Logic would dictate that the cause of the dementia, whatever it might be, is pursued later. It is for this reason primarily that it is urged that the misnomer 'pseudo-dementia' be dropped (Mahendra, 1983). When depression appears to be a key clinical feature and the probable cause of the dementia, the term 'dementia syndrome of depression' (Folstein and McHugh, 1978) has been suggested.

An appreciation of this conceptual basis to the diagnosis of dementia will also help clear up the confusion surrounding the findings of several workers (Kendell, 1974; Nott and Fleminger, 1975; Ron et al., 1979) who have bemoaned the high proportion of 'erroneous' diagnoses. If a patient displays the features of dementia over a sustained period of time he is demented, whatever else he might have or turn out to be. The case history in Chapter 2 illustrates this point.

The proportion of dementias due to a depression and other psychiatric illnesses will vary according to the kind of institution receiving the patient. Two dissimilar institutions (Marsden and Harrison, 1972; Smith and Kiloh, 1981) seemed to attract between 10% and 15% depressive and psychiatric cases among the pre-senile dements. In the latter study the proportion dropped considerably among patients who were over 65 years old, who presumably were more susceptible to Alzheimer's disease. This would imply that the eminently treatable depressive dementia must be sought for most assiduously amongst younger patients.

We may take this opportunity to consider the assumptions regarding the concept of 'pseudo-dementia'. The idea that a reversible dementia induced by depression (which is only the commonest among several 'functional' causes of reversible dementia) exists has not been seriously disputed. The mechanism usually put forward to argue for a depression-induced dementia is as follows. Changes following upon a depressive illness in an elderly person impinge on a brain affected by the changes of normal ageing – and perhaps functioning at borderline levels of activity – and help nudge it into a state which manifests clinically as dementia. Thus the idea of a 'threshold' – also used to explain the onset of dementia in Alzheimer's disease and multi-infarct vascular disease – is entertained. Since depressive illness occurs most frequently in and beyond middle age, when structural brain changes of ageing are found to be significantly greater than in the younger subject, the scope for a 'pseudo-dementing' presentation was accordingly so much greater in the elderly depressed patient. The crux of this concept of 'pseudo-dementia' was that when the depression was treated and reversed, the cognitive changes subsided and the dementia receded with no apparent sequelae.

Let us now consider the evidence. For a start, far from being synonymous with depression-induced dementia, 'pseudo-dementia' appears in association with several psychiatric conditions. Mania, hysteria, drug toxicity, schizophrenia, thyrotoxicosis, hypochondriasis and paranoid illness are some of the conditions noted in the literature. Also, while anecdotal and single case reports suggest it is the elderly who present with 'pseudo-dementia', the evidence from reported series of cases seems to suggest a wider range. Wells (1979) gave an age range between 33 and 69, and said seven of his ten patients were in their fifties or sixties. Smith and Kiloh (1981), reporting a series of 200 demented patients of all ages, showed that 'pseudo-dementia' accounted for 10% of all dementias under 45 years and 13.6% of dementias between the ages of 45 and 64 years, but only for 1.8% of dementias over 65 years. McAllister's (1983) pooled series of cases yielded a mean of 60.5 years with a range between 22 and 85 years. Marsden and Harrison (1972), Nott and Fleminger (1975) and Ron et al. (1979) all paid attention to pre-senile cases of dementia with significant numbers of 'pseudo-dements', with Ron et al. (1979) commenting that 'pseudo-dementia' was underemphasized in younger age groups. Thus the prevalence of 'depressive pseudo-dementia' in relatively young patients, when by prediction it should have been found with increasing frequency in the patient in whom depression obtrudes upon the brain changes of ageing, needs to be explained. Also, while it is true, as Tomlinson et al. (1968) have shown, that structural brain changes in non-demented old people increase with age – in effect producing a closer approximation to Alzheimer-like pathology than in the younger subject – there is no difference between changes in the brain between such non-dementing conditions as physical illness, confusional states, depressive illness and paraphrenia (Tomlinson et al., 1968; Roth, 1980). Thus, there is no especially susceptible brain available in the patient with depressive illness to be urged beyond a threshold into dementia. The fact that depressive 'pseudo-dementia' occurs in middle age and not necessarily, or preferentially, in the senium, when age changes make the brain most vulnerable, suggests there is more to 'pseudo-dementia' than the fortuitous association between depressive illness and the ageing brain.

Furthermore, if 'pseudo-dementia' was indeed induced simply by depression, it would be expected that the depressed affect would precede cognitive change and there might be a time interval between the onset of depression and the onset of dementia. But this does not seem to occur invariably. Clinical experience bears out that depression and dementia often have a simultaneous onset. The lack of a consistent temporal relationship between affective and cognitive change is matched by an inconsistent quantitative relationship. Very often, memory difficulties are seen to be as prominent as, if not more so than, the depressive features. McAllister and Price (1982) noted a profound degree of cognitive impairment which appeared to be greatly out of proportion to the degree of depressive symptoms.

In fact, with the modern management of depressive illness it is unlikely that depression will be allowed to reach a late stage at which dementia emerged.

As Shraberg (1978) and McAllister et al. (1982) showed, even when the depression of a 'depressive pseudo-dementia' is removed by treatment, the dementia does not automatically recede. It is, in fact, a not uncommon observation that a full recovery from depression is not reflected in corresponding progress in the course of the dementia. Further, one would expect, if indeed the syndrome of dementia in these cases were merely an extension of the depressive illness, the manifest brain changes in 'pseudo-dementia' not to exceed those to be found in depressive, or other functional psychiatric, illness. But Wells (1979) revealed that half of his 'pseudo-dements' seemed to have some evidence of brain damage. Nott and Fleminger (1975) noted evidence of organic impairment on psychometry, cortical atrophy on air encephalographic studies and abnormality in the EEG in a larger than expected proportion of 'pseudo-dements'. McAllister (1983) remarked that the status of EEG findings in cases of 'pseudo-dementia' was uncertain, whereas, as it is widely acknowledged, the EEG changes in depression and other 'functional' disorders are non-specific enough to be disregarded in ordinary practice.

All in all, we have an altogether more complex situation than the idea of 'pseudo-dementia' induced and sustained by depression and dependent on its course for its own symptomatology. If the concept of 'pseudo-dementia' is untenable in terms of logic, and misleading in clinical practice, the facts regarding its other properties are even more emphatic. The wise course for the present would be to speak of 'dementia associated with depression' or the 'dementia syndrome of depression'.

The clinical features of depression and other psychiatric illness associated with the syndrome of dementia are probably best appreciated in relation to the presentation of the more usual forms of dementia. Table 3.4 is modified from Wells (1979) to show the distinction between depressive dementia and Alzheimer's disease.

The term 'pseudo-dementia' seems more applicable to three other states of psychiatric causation. In the intriguing Ganser Syndrome, described originally by Ganser (1898; trans. 1965) as 'A Peculiar Hysterical State', the essential feature of the syndrome is usually described as *Vorbeireden* (to talk at cross purposes), though it has been suggested that *Vorbeigehen* (to pass

55

by) might be a more accurate description. Here the patient makes wrong, and often ridiculously wrong, responses to simple questions yet reveals by the tone of the answer that the intent of the question was clear to him. In one of Ganser's cases the following exchange took place between interviewer and patient:

> 'How many legs does a horse have?'
> 'Three.'
> 'An elephant?'
> 'Five.'
> 'What follows one?'
> 'Two.'
> 'Then?'
> 'Twelve, ninety-three.'

Anderson and Mallison (1941) made it clear that any random or approximate answer did not qualify, and suggested the definition as

> That false response of a patient to the examiner's question where the answer, although wrong, is never far wrong and bears a definite and obvious relation to the question, indicating clearly the question has been grasped by the patient.

Ganser's other invariable features of the syndrome were that the patients were undoubtedly ill (and not simulating madness), had strong hysterical stigmata, fluctuating clouding of consciousness, defects of memory and hallucinations, and all were precipitated by physical or emotional trauma. Whether the condition amounts to dementia is arguable, for clouding of consciousness is invariable and the apparent intellectual deficit is incomplete and changeable.

At the time of Ganser's paper, and for some years afterwards, it was believed that Ganser syndrome existed largely, if not exclusively, among the prison population. It is a rare condition now and a distinction is drawn between the Ganser state and the symptoms which may appear in schizophrenia, depression and other psychoses, following head injury, alcoholism and in the early stages of dementia. The Ganser state or symptom is of brief duration and ends spontaneously, often leaving an amnesia for the episode.

Another variant, also in arguable relationship to dementia, is what has been called *hysterical pseudo-dementia*. Here, a suggestible and somewhat backward individual, who might occasionally have a history of conversion symptoms in the past, responds to some emotional trauma by becoming demented in the sense that there is gross memory disturbance and an incapacity to respond to elementary questions or commands or situations. Very often, in an institutional setting, they may settle into an existence which is physically adequate though the mental changes continue being gross. The mood is one of bland indifference though a superficial theatricality of manner can also be observed. The course the episode runs depends on the patient's rather vulnerable personality, and even upon recovery the chance of relapse must be put high.

Whether a category of *simulated dementia* exists is highly debatable.

Ovid (43 BC–AD 17) had said, 'He who can counterfeit sanity will be sane', and it is the impression of most clinicians that a convincing simulation of dementia cannot be sustained for more than a very short period and that persistent inquiry will reveal the true state. As with hysterical pseudo-

Table 3.4 The distinction between depressive dysfunction and Alzheimer's disease (modified after Wells, 1979).

'Depressive dementia'	Alzheimer's disease
Clinical course	
1. Onset can be dated with some precision.	1. Onset dated only within broad limits.
2. Symptoms of relatively short duration.	2. Symptoms of longer duration before medical help sought.
3. History of previous psychiatric illness of similar kind common.	3. Previous psychiatric history unusual.
4. Relatively rapid progression of symptoms after onset.	4. Slow progression of symptoms throughout course.
5. Family usually very aware of the dysfunction and its severity.	5. Family usually unaware of the dysfunction and its severity.
Clinical features	
1. Patients complain much of cognitive loss.	1. Patients complain little of cognitive loss.
2. Patients make detailed complaints of cognitive dysfunction.	2. Complaints usually vague.
3. Patients emphasize disability.	3. Patients conceal disability.
4. Patients highlight failure.	4. Patients delight in accomplishments, however trivial.
5. Patients make little effort to perform even simple tasks.	5. Patients struggle to perform tasks.
6. Patients do not try to keep up.	6. Patients rely on notes, diaries and calendar to keep up.
7. Patients usually communicate strong sense of distress.	7. Patients often appear unconcerned.
8. There is pervasive affective change.	8. Affect labile and shallow.
9. Nocturnal accentuation of dysfunction uncommon.	9. Nocturnal accentuation common.
Features of cognitive dysfunction	
1. 'Don't know' answers typical.	1. 'Near miss' and wrong answers frequent.
2. Memory gaps for specific periods of events common.	2. Memory gaps for specific periods unusual.
3. Marked variability in performing tasks of similar difficulty.	3. Consistently poor performance on tasks of similar difficulty.

dementia the cognitive impairment on clinical examination is often out of keeping with the behaviour of the patient when he is not observed, and he may go about the rest of his business in the most adequate fashion. On a hospital ward populated by sick patients it is usually striking how little physical attention needs to be paid to the person simulating dementia or other serious mental illness. However, the distinction between conscious simulation and illness (including hysterical behaviour) is not easy, being dependent on impressions about motivation that have to be assessed by the clinician who in turn has his own motives – ideological, philosophical or political – in coming to a conclusion. It has been suggested that if, in the absence of obvious dissease, a person gives the impression of knowing what he is doing and why he is doing it, he is probably simulating. A practical test which is used with some success on psychiatric wards is to challenge the patient. The hysterical patient may be indifferent to persistent questioning and carry on as before. The person simulating illness becomes angry and defensive and tends to become very suspicious and cautious in his behaviour in the presence of his inquisitors.

THE HYDROCEPHALIC DEMENTIAS

The causes of dementing illness associated with hydrocephalus are several. Table 3.5 below is a brief list.

Table 3.5   Some possible causes of hydrocephalic dementias (after Benson, 1975)

Non-obstructive		
Degenerative	–	Alzheimer's disease, Pick's disease, senile dementias of unidentified origin
Destructive	–	Arteriosclerotic, traumatic dementias
Obstructive		
Non-communicating	–	Ventricular obstruction
Communicating	–	Normal pressure hydrocephalus
Other		
Cerebral cyst		
Ectatic basilar artery		

The condition of special interest to us is the syndrome of normal pressure hydrocephalus (NPH) which was defined by Hakim and Adams in 1965. Clinically, the presentation is with gait disturbance, dementia and incontinence. Radiologically there is massive hydrocephalus despite free communication between the ventricular system and the lumber subarachnoid space, with a normal cerebrospiral fluid pressure. Therapeutically, there often is improvement following a shunt of excess cerebrospinal fluid.

There are two forms of NPH. The first is a form that occurs secondary to lesions which may produce a communicating or obstructive hydrocephalus. About two-thirds of all patients with NPH have a prior history of subarachnoid haemorrhage, head trauma or meningitis. Approximately 60% of these patients show definite improvement after shunting procedures (Katzman, 1976, 1978).

The other form is the 'idiopathic NPH' brought to prominence by Adams *et al.* (1965). The aetiology of this condition is obviously uncertain but suggestions have included low-grade asymptomatic inflammatory meningeal disease, arachnoid thickening and vascular disease. An unexpectedly high incidence of hypertensive cerebrovascular disease has been found at autopsy in patients who had been diagnosed in life as 'idiopathic NPH' (Katzman, 1978). A favourable response to shunting is seen in only 40% of cases of this type.

It appears to be a disease of the pre-senium and the incidence of idiopathic NPH among patients with pre-senile dementia is considerably (some 20–30 times) greater than in senile dementia.

Despite the presence of the triad of gait disturbance, dementia and incontinence, the diagnosis, and the differentiation from Alzheimer's disease, is not always clear-cut, as some 10% of patients with Alzheimer's disease may have severely dilated ventricles and satisfy the radiological criteria for the diagnosis of NPH (Katzman, 1978). However, the points of distinction in the average case are clear. Where Alzheimer's disease invariably begins with memory and intellectual difficulties NPH has as its first symptom gait disturbance. This is characterized by a slow, unsteady gait in which the feet act as if they are magnetized to the floor. The gait changes in Alzheimer's disease occur later in the illness. Confusion is more likely to occur with the 'lacunar state' gait changes. Moreover, patients with Alzheimer's disease, even when they show clinical and radiological changes of NPH, do not respond to shunting.

Arteriography, which shows bowing of the arterior cerebral artery, lateral displacement of the sylvian vessels and displacement of the thalamostriate veins, may be suggestive but the characteristic picture emerges on cisternography. There is immediate isotope concentration in the ventricles where it may remain for 48–72 hours. There is little or no movement of isotope into the cortical arachnoid space and to the sagittal region (Benson, 1975).

Gustafson and Hagberg (1978), considering the response of a mixed group of patients to ventriculo-atrial shunt procedures, reported that an acute onset and a clinical picture dominated by memory difficulty predicted a good outcome after shunt operation. The best therapeutic effect was seen in those with a well-defined syndrome of hydrocephalic dementia with symptoms such as confabulation, gait disturbance, urinary incontinence, lack of insight and constructional apraxia. These symptoms, they felt, might only be incidental or associated findings. When it came to aetiological factors those patients who showed most improvement seemed to have had subarachnoid haemorrhage, obstructional hydrocephalus and previous intracranial operation while those with 'idiopathic' hydrocephalus and skull trauma, often with associated alcoholism, improved least.

The pathology of the condition is uncertain but the gait disturbance is attributed to a lesion in the long fibre tracts in the periventricular tissue, a site also affected in the lacunar state. Dementia and urinary incontinence have also been found in the lacunar state and it would not be surprising if the two conditions came to share some common elements. A further point in favour of some vascular involvement in idiopathic NPH is the suggestion that shunt procedures improve the clinical state not only by relieving the distension of ventricles and the stasis of cerebrospinal fluid with its stale metabolites but by correcting a loss of autoregulation in cerebral blood flow.

DEMENTIAS DUE TO TRAUMA

Two conditions of a dissimilar kind, but united in the capacity to manifest dementia months and years after injury has been inflicted on the head, must now be considered.

Subdural haematoma

In this condition blood collects in the subdural space following rupture of veins. This usually follows head injury, though it may occasionally arise in those on anticoagulants or with bleeding diathesis. The history of head injury is not always obtained, partly because the course of the illness is subacute or chronic. In the usual type of presentation a marked feature is the fluctuating level of consciousness from day to day. The mental state varies correspondingly with impaired concentration, lapses of memory and reduced mentation.

It is the more chronic form of the condition which is confused with dementia, especially in the elderly and when the head injury is missed. The memory difficulties become more pronounced and the intellectual failure becomes well established.

The investigation of the condition in the early stages has been revolutionized by computerized tomography but in the chronic, long-standing form of the illness results of surgical intervention remain poor and the residual dementia can be severe.

Martland in 1928 drew attention to the 'punch-drunk' state in boxers, in which experienced boxers, after retirement, became unsteady, forgetful and physically and mentally slow. Roberts (1969) surveyed 224 ex-professional boxers and found a clinical syndrome in 17% of them. This syndrome included deficiencies in intellect and memory, and a neurological dys-function involving pyramidal, extrapyramidal and cerebellar pathways. Corsellis *et al.* (1973) studied 15 cases, 12 of whom showed some serious abnormality of movement such as tremor, ataxia or dysarthria. There was hemiparesis, and roughly half the number had become excessively sensitive to small quantities of alcohol. There was physical and mental deterioration and eight of them had died in psychiatric institutions.

Corsellis (1978) has considered the neuropathological findings which are appropriately dealt with here. He has discussed them under the headings of

(1) septal and hypothalamic anomalies;
(2) cerebellar lesions;
(3) degeneration of the substantia nigra;
(4) occurrence of Alzheimer's neurofibrillary tangles in the absence of neuritic plaques. This change is concentrated in the limbic grey matter and is indistinguishable from the changes of Alzheimer's disease.

Corsellis believes the neuropathological picture in this form of post-traumatic injury leading to dementia is distinctive, and rules out most other known neuropathologies such as alcoholism and cerebral syphilis. The relationship with Alzheimer's disease is a curious one but the changes in septum, hypothalamus, cerebellum and the substantia nigra are not seen in the typical case of Alzheimer's disease. One explanation might be that repeated, skilfully applied blows to the head cause lesions in parts of the brain vulnerable to attack and at the same time predispose to an Alzheimer-like change in other parts.

SUBCORTICAL DEMENTIA

In this chapter up to now the assumption has been that, in a case of 'organic' dementia with discernible brain pathology, the lesion is to be found in the cerebral cortex. In the 1920s Van Bogaert and Bertrand described a syndrome due to subacute degeneration of brain stem structures and the cerebellum, which led to dementia. Over the years lesions of the globus pallidus, pons, cerebellum and the thalamus have been shown occasionally to lead to dementia in the apparent absence of cortical involvement. Gascon and Gilles (1973) reported a case of selective, but complete, limbic lobe destruction which ended with dementia, with a severe amnestic syndrome with confabulation, a Kluver Bucy-like syndrome and personality change, which they suggested could be called 'limbic dementia'. However, it has to be said that intellectual deterioration could not be established in their patient and the possibility exists that clinically theirs was a variant of the dysmnesic syndrome.

Albert (1978), who has given a concise account of the subcortical dementias, states the term refers to a behavioural syndrome found in patients with a variety of neurological illnesses in which prominent pathological changes are seen in subcortical nuclear structures (e.g. progressive supranuclear palsy, Parkinson's disease, Huntington's chorea). Clinically this syndrome manifests itself by

(1) emotional or personality changes, typically inertia or apathy, occasionally with brief outbursts of anger;
(2) memory disorder;
(3) defective ability to manipulate acquired knowledge;
(4) marked slowness in the rate of information processing.

The subcortical dementias may be contrasted clinically with the more usual cortical dementias with pathological changes in the cerebral cortex. In the subcortical dementias, vocabulary and language function are generally preserved. One effect of this might be a failure to register intellectual deterioration on a vocabulary-based intelligence test. Parietal lobe dysfunction in the form of aphasia, apraxia and agnosia is also not seen in the subcortical dementias. In the cortical dementias, however, aphasia, agnosia and apraxia are seen in combination with the features of dementia.

It has also been pointed out that the symptom complex of subcortical dementia is similar to the behavioural syndrome seen in patients with frontal lobe damage. As there is a link between the frontal cortex and the limbic system and its subcortical connections, the term 'fronto-limbic dementia' has also been suggested.

The dementia of Huntington's chorea has already been discussed and a few words need to be said about the dementia of Parkinson's disease. Impairment of intellectual function amounting to dementia in this condition has been found in 20–40% of patients (Mindham *et al.*, 1982). Dementia is rarely an early feature, more often occurring after 5 years of treatment (Marsden, 1982). There is some dispute as to the mechanism. Marsden (1982) has argued that a superimposed Alzheimer's disease might be the cause of dementia but this is denied by Perry *et al.* (1983), who have suggested that reduced cholinergic activities in Parkinson's disease usually occur in the absence of Alzheimer's disease (as defined in conventional histopathological terms). A way of reconciling this difference of opinion is discussed in Chapter 8.

It must also be stated that though depression is a common feature of Parkinson's disease, considerably more patients are depressed than demented in this condition, and the relationship between them is less significant than it might appear.

DEMENTIA DUE TO ALCOHOLISM

This is a vexed problem. Apart from the intrinsic difficulty in ascertaining the role of a substance which is used and abused to such a considerable extent, the writings on the subject of alcohol and dementia have not served to clarify the issue. Victor and Banker (1978) have given a comprehensive review under the title of 'Alcohol and Dementia', but in their dementias they include the Wernicke-Korsakoff syndrome, which is characterized by a severe dysmnesic syndrome rather than by dementia, and hepatic encephalopathy. This is a controversial classification and is at odds with the concept of dementia as understood in this country.

Lishman's (1981) remarks on alcoholic dementia in his survey of cerebral syndromes of impairment in alcoholism is more representative. He has referred to historical descriptions which tend to show that a concept of alcoholic dementia, in terms that we would understand, abounded in the 19th-century literature but after the introduction of the term Korsakoff syndrome in the early part of this century, clinicians seemed to prefer the use of the newer term. Lishman wonders if the former dements have now become improperly labelled.

Epidemiological evidence is lacking for the incidence of dementia due to alcoholism, but Lishman (1981) quotes three surveys from the UK, Australia and the USA on hospitalized patients in which alcohol had been suspected as a cause in a substantial proportion of dements, approximately as frequently as multi-infarct dementia. There is also evidence from psychologists about the cognitive impairment in alcoholics, from neuropathologists about histological lesions and from radiologists about cortical atrophy on air studies and on computerized tomography. These seem to be consistent findings and are of interest in themselves but they do not amount to dementia in terms of the definitions in current use.

A more revealing study, which throws some light on the over-emphasis on the diagnosis of the Wernicke-Korsakoff psychosis, is by Cutting (1978) who retrospectively studied 50 alcoholics diagnosed as Korsakoff's psychosis and 13 who had been called alcoholic dements. When he subdivided his Korsakoff group into those with illness of acute onset and those with gradual onset, he found the latter approximated closely to the 'dementia' group in terms of sex, age, duration of symptoms, psychometric change and subsequent improvement. This group, despite the generally pessimistic connotation of the term 'dementia', also did considerably better than those with acute-onset Korsakoff's psychosis. It seemed that the suspicion that alcoholic dementias were being admitted under some other diagnostic categories was well based. It is not, however, clear if this is the only category of alcoholic dementia, and it is possible that alcoholics at a later stage in their lives and their drinking careers will have a less reversible condition and a poorer prognosis.

DEMENTIA ASSOCIATED WITH MALIGNANT DISEASE

Brain and Henson's (1958) concept of paraneoplastic disorder would take account of dementia occurring in the presence of neoplastic disease elsewhere in the body and without discernible cause. It is not the commonest mental manifestation of neoplastic disease. Depression comes first and although organic change comes next, it is usually in the form of clouding of consciousness or delirium. Among the explanations given for the appearance of dementia in malignant disease are metastatic deposits, infiltrations, specific nutritional disorder, ectopic hormone production and other metabolic disorders, infections, including progressive multifocal leucoencephalopathy, and the unwanted effects of treatment (Henson and Urich, 1982).

GENERAL PARESIS

This condition, which filled hospital wards in the early 19th century, is now a rarity but its historical importance and protean manifestations ('He who knows syphilis knows medicine') make a brief account imperative.

Males were more commonly affected than females, the peak age of onset being middle age, some 20 years or so from the time of the primary infection.

Dementia is a relatively late feature and the disease usually presents after a non-specific prodromal stage with memory difficulties, personality change or depression. The memory deficit goes hand in hand with intellectual deterioration, whereas the personality change may suggest frontal lobe involvement.

The well-known grandiose form of the illness is now rare, accounting for only 10% of Dewhurst's (1969) series. More commonly the illness presents with depression or simple dementia and these seem to account for nearly 50% of presentations. A combined picture of tabes dorsalis and general paresis may be seen in another 20% of cases.

The pupillary changes including the well-known Argyll-Robertson pupil

63

are found in about 70% of cases, and optic atrophy may also present. A coarse irregular tremor involving the hands and face is found in about two-thirds of cases. Dysarthria is another common feature, as are abnormalities in reflexes and in gait.

The diagnosis, which may be suspected on a positive venereal disease research laboratory (VDRL) test, is confirmed by the *Treponema pallidum* immobilization (TPI) test or the flourescent treponemal antibody (FTA) test. The blood yields positive results in 90% of cases but the cerebrospinal fluid is thought always to be affected and yields positive serology. The Lange colloidal gold curve gives a paretic curve with a first zone rise.

METABOLIC DEMENTIAS

It is customary for writers to provide long lists of metabolic causes of dementia even though many alleged aetiological processes have not been established to produce the changes in intellect, memory and personality to satisfy the requirements of the definition. It is very likely that many of the agents and processes usually mentioned, including drugs, cause a disturbance of consciousness with the occcasional delirium. Roth (1982), as we have noted, has emphasized this point further. To repeat, the brain, he has said, is well insulated from the adverse metabolic effects of most forms of extracerebral disease and if chronic respiratory, cardiovascular, hepatic and renal disease cause any psychiatric complication they almost invariably give rise to a subacute, fluctuating, clouded or delirious state. He feels the same about pernicious anaemia and other toxic and deficiency diseases that are given in lists.

A good case in point would be *dialysis dementia*, a syndrome first described in 1972 which has as its hallmarks progressive speech difficulties, altered sensorium and a markedly abnormal EEG with other features frequently seen being epileptic seizures, myoclonus, asterixis, apraxia and psychosis. Though a growing literature since that time has described the condition as a dementia it would be more appropriate to classify it among the toxic confusional states.

Interestingly, when formal surveys of the causes of dementia are undertaken one finds the incidence of metabolic causes is less than 1% (Plum, 1978). It seems that when diagnostic criteria are applied with some rigour the mental manifestations are not deemed to amount to dementia.

Plum (1978) has also indicated those metabolic causes which may be 'especially prone to produce irreversible cerebral injury and dementia'. His list includes Wilson's disease, thiamine and niacin deficiency, selective industrial hydrocarbon and heavy metal toxicity, hyperinsulinism and chronic dialysis-induced dementia. The arguments put forward earlier would still prevail. The logical course in a case with metabolic disturbance and dementia would be to assess the changes separately and to seek a causal relationship with scepticism. As a general rule, prompt treatment of the metabolic change is advocated.

SUMMARY

(1) The classification of the dementias must at present be partly descriptive and partly aetiological.

(2) It is also possible that conditions that appear clinically homogeneous may with time come to be seen as collections of different disorders, with dementia being merely a common end-point.

(3) *Alzheimer's disease* is probably the commonest cause of senile and pre-senile dementia. It is commoner among females and has an uncertain genetic basis. Three stages of the illness can be noted. The first shows memory difficulty and the progression is insidious. Depression is a feature of this stage. The second stage manifests parietal lobe symptoms and intellectual deterioration and personality change are also observed. The third and terminal stage is marked by severe neurological disability, incontinence and emaciation. The course runs between 2 and 5 years. The younger patient shows a more serious affliction, may be one of an affected family group and shows more marked parietal, and possibly temporal, lobe involvement with florid neurological phenomena.

(4) The *vascular dementias* include 'arteriosclerotic' and multi-infarct dementias. Variants include the 'lacunar state' and subcortical arteriosclerotic encephalopathy (Binswanger's disease). There has almost certainly been an over-diagnosis of vascular dementia because elderly normal brains at autopsy have shown cerebral infarctions. There is no convincing relationship between disease in the larger arteries in the neck and dementia. There are several causes including hypertensive arterial disease and cardiovascular disease leading to thrombo-embolic phenomena. In the common variety of the disease the sex difference is in favour of slightly higher male involvement. The onset is relatively sudden and a feature of the illness is a progression by fits and starts or 'step-wise'. The clinical features which have been traditionally used to separate this dementia from Alzheimer's disease and other non-vascular dementias have been put into the Hachinski Ischaemic Score. Survival is somewhat longer than in Alzheimer's disease. The lacunar state and Binswanger's disease have been described.

(5) *Pick's disease* is commoner in women and autosomal dominant transmission has been implicated. It is a pre-senile dementia. Frontal lobe involvement with marked personality change is a common early feature. There is a sparing of constructional and visuo-spatial ability but an earlier speech deficit than in Alzheimer's disease. Periods of survival may be up to 10 years.

(6) *Huntington's chorea* occurs equally in both sexes and is thought to be due to autosomal dominant transmission. The age of onset is variable but usually between 35 and 40 years. Behavioural changes,

including florid psychiatric syndromes, come first, to be followed by chorea and dementia. The impact of the mental changes on family life can be serious. Suicide is common. The period of survival is about 15 years, though in childhood the illness runs a much shorter course. The variations of the disorder among children and young adults have been described.

(7) *Creutzfeldt–Jakob disease* occurs in both men and women to a similar extent and occasional familial cases have been described. A great variety of neurological symptomatology is seen, and this precedes the changes of dementia. It is a rapidly progressing illness and most patients are dead within 2 years. Some of the variants of the classical picture such as the amyotrophic, subacute spongiform and cerebellar forms are described.

(8) *'Pseudo-dementia'* is usually taken to refer to those cases of dementia of presumed functional psychiatric origin. The logical and practical objection to the term is discussed. Depressive illness is by far the commonest 'cause' of this form of dementia and may account for up to 15% of all cases of dementia. An attempt has been made to show that the distinction between depressive dementia and any other dementia is with regard to the respective causes of the syndrome. The Ganser state, hysterical pseudo-dementia and simulated dementia, which have a better claim to be called 'pseudo-dementias', are discussed.

(9) The *hydrocephalic dementias* include idiopathic normal pressure hydrocephalus which was described in 1965. About 40–60% of these patients respond to surgery. It is primarily a cause of pre-senile dementia and is characterized in addition by gait disturbance and incontinence. It has some pathological affiliations with vascular dementia.

(10) Two important post-traumatic dementias are *subdural haematoma* and the chronic encephalopathy seen in boxers after retirement. Chronic subdural haematoma in the elderly leads to serious diagnostic confusion and the outcome, even after the condition is detected, is grave. In the 'punch-drunk' syndrome, retired professional boxers show neurological dysfunction and dementia. There are definite, and probably distinctive, neuropathological changes, and the presence of neurofibrillary tangles, although in the absence of neuritic plaques, raises the possibility of some relationship to the histological changes of Alzheimer's disease.

(11) In the *subcortical dementias* the syndrome of dementia appears to be present in the absence of significant pathology in the cerebral cortex. Lesions in the globus pallidus, pons, cerebellum and thalamus have been noted in this condition. Dementias associated with Huntington's chorea, Parkinson's disease and progressive supranuclear palsy are sometimes traced to subcortical lesions. A cardinal feature is the

preservation of language and parietal lobe function. In view of postulated links between the frontal lobe and the limbic system the term 'fronto-limbic dementia' has also been suggested for this condition.

(12) *Alcoholic dementia* is a somewhat controversial entity because the term dementia has been used loosely in relation to mental changes in alcoholism and also because changes in diagnostic fashion seem to have accounted for cases of dementia under other categories and led to an apparent decline in the prevalence of cases. In formal surveys, however, the condition is not uncommon. It now appears that some of the cases of gradually progressing Korsakoff's psychosis can be considered on clinical and psychometric grounds to be cases of alcoholic dementia.

(13) Dementias associated with malignant disease are not common but they are one form of paraneoplastic disorder.

(14) General paresis is now a rarity. It occurs about 20 years after the primary infection and affects men more frequently. The common presentation nowadays is with depression or a simple dementing illness. Classical neurological signs are seen and modern immuno-logical tests make a firm diagnosis possible.

(15) Dementias due to metabolic dysfunction and drug toxicity are probably less common than it is thought, and it has been suggested the confusion may have arisen because of the disturbances of consciousness these processes and agents undeniably cause. When strict criteria are applied in formal surveys of dementing illness the contribution from these causes is usually seen to be less than 1%. The much-publicized dialysis dementia is a case in point.

Further reading

(A full list of references is given at the end of the book.)

Katzman, R., Terry, R.D. and Bick, K.L. (eds) (1978). *Alzheimer's Disease: Senile Dementia and Related Disorders.* (New York: Raven Press)

Lishman, W.A. (1978). Senile dementia, presenile dementia and pseudodementia. In *Organic Psychiatry.* (London: Blackwell)

Office of Health Economics (1980). *Huntington's Chorea.* (London)

Ropper, A.H. (1979). A rational approach to dementia. *Can. Med. Assoc. J.*, **121**, 1175-1188

Roth, M. (1980). Senile dementia and its borderlands. In Cole, J.O. and Barrett, J.E. (eds) *Psychopathology in the Aged.* (New York: Raven Press)

Roth, M. (1982). Perspectives in the diagnosis of senile and pre-senile dementia of Alzheimer type. In Sarner, M. (ed.) *Advanced Medicine*, **Vol. 18.** (London: the Royal College of Physicians and Pitman Medical)

4
Psychological testing in dementia

Measure your mind's height by the shade it casts:
Robert Browning (1812–1889)

The role of psychometry is to assess in quantitative terms the behavioural changes that might be found in patients. The term behaviour when applied to demented patients refers largely to aspects of intellectual and memory function. As might be expected in an area so very individual, the measurement of personality function, and more particularly dysfunction, is far from satisfactory for general clinical purposes.

The concept of dementia has been discussed at length in Chapter 2, where it was emphasized repeatedly that the diagnosis, in the present state of knowledge, is a clinical matter. Patients do not present as demented to clinicians but come with complaints suggestive of deteriorating intellectual function, impaired memory and changed (usually for the worse and apparent in many instances only to friends and near relatives) personality, and the clinician satisfies himself that they fit the criteria for the dementia syndrome. The clinician then refers the patient to a psychologist who is invited to contribute usually to three areas in which the clinician is primarily interested:

(1) Quantification, i.e. putting figures to, and establishing a baseline for future reference of, those changes detected in the clinical assessment of intellectual and memory function.

(2) Testing and measuring areas of specific dysfunction in the patient's behaviour which might provide further information towards a differential diagnosis and clues to a possible aetiology. This is analogous to the role played by laboratory investigation and is further taken up below.

(3) Measuring and establishing the areas of preserved function so that

69

while the patient's disabilities are recorded, a note is made of his strengths and abilities which are made use of in management and basic rehabilitation.

It is necessary to be realistic about the limitations of psychometric assessment. Lishman (1978) has provided a clear, concise account of the role of the clinical psychologist in organic psychiatry. When it comes to dementia, it must be plain that it is necessary to interpret psychometric test results in conjunction with clinical and other laboratory data. As Lishman puts it, no single test will differentiate brain-damaged patients from others without some degree of overlap, and reliance on these tests alone is likely to produce misleading information.

The reason given by Lishman for this is that in their standardization, tests might have been employed on clear-cut cases whereas clinicians seek out special psychometric assistance when they are most in doubt. As we have repeatedly stressed, the diagnosis of dementia is based on clinical criteria but the 'final arbiter' of the cause of a dementing process is pathology and psychometric evaluation is at the same disadvantage as are all other investigatory procedures.

As was shown in Chapters 2 and 3, dementia can present with a variety of deficits. Thus tests which sample a restricted aspect of cognitive activity may fail to identify other, sufficiently circumscribed cerebral lesions. Purely verbal tests, for example, may fail to detect visuospatial deficits resulting from a lesion of the non-dominant hemisphere. Even with diffuse brain damage the behavioural effects which follow may vary at different levels of functional disorganization, so that tests which tap one hierarchical level of behaviour may fail entirely to tap another (Lishman, 1978).

A blunderbuss approach to testing, when an enormous range of functions are tested by a battery, will result in general cover but will lack the sensitivity to strike small, barely noticeable areas of cognitive dysfunction that may lurk within more restricted areas of brain activity.

However, when the psychologist with his tests becomes an ally of the clinician, the partnership can become a considerably more powerful one. The clinician has the advantage that he is the arbiter of the diagnosis but the psychologist has as his stock-in-trade standardized tests which are numerically scored. Norms have been laboriously worked out, can now be read off tables and applied to the behaviour of the individual patient. Also these tests can be repeated with the expectation of reliable results even in the hands of another psychologist at another institution. Equivocal findings can be confirmed and the first readings can always be used as a base or a frame of reference.

Psychologists also have another advantage over the conventional clinician in that they can concentrate in greater detail on single areas of suspected dysfunction. The range of psychological tests is vast and even though only a few that we shall presently describe are used as first-line tests, several others are available as reserves and can be brought into play if a specific need arises. In this way minor memory or dysphasic difficulties can be explored in greater detail.

The principle upon which neuropsychological testing and interpretation are based is essentially a simple one. It is assumed that verbal and symbolic activity is a function of the parts of the dominant (usually the left) hemisphere and temporal and visuospatial activity is dependent on the non-dominant (usually the right) hemisphere. Left parietal lobe lesions, for example, are associated with difficulties with arithmetic, digit span and sentence learning: right parietal lesions with picture arrangement and memory for designs. On the tests of learning and retention the impairment obviously depends on the nature of the test material – verbal material is mainly affected by left-sided lesions (especially left temporal) and visual material by right-sided lesions (particularly right parietal).

SOME PSYCHOMETRIC TESTS USED ON DEMENTED PATIENTS

The Wechsler Adult Intelligence Scale (WAIS)

This test has been available since 1944 and is used for the measurement of intelligence, providing separate scores for verbal and performance abilities. It is possible to assess deterioration from the premorbid level, usually estimated, and the standardized sub-test scores can be individually studied.

There are 11 sub-tests in the complete WAIS battery.

Verbal sub-tests
1. Information: Questions cover a range of general information.
2. Comprehension: Tests common sense and judgement.
3. Arithmetic: Tests simple arithmetical knowledge.
4. Similarities: Tests which require the similarities between things to be explained.
5. Digit span: Lists of digits to be reproduced forwards and backwards.
6. Vocabulary: Tests ability to give meanings of words.

Performance sub-tests
1. Digit symbol: Tests ability to match symbols to digits.
2. Picture completion: Tests ability of subject to complete missing details of picture.
3. Block design: Tests ability to reproduce designs with test blocks.
4. Picture arrangement: Tests ability to arrange a set of cards so as to tell a story.
5. Object assembly: Tests ability to assemble objects from their individual parts.

A score is obtained on each test and is converted into a standard score and details of the mean and variation of each test are available for comparison. The standardized scores may be compared one with another.

The significant score in patients with dementia is thought to be the deterioration index which is derived from 'Hold tests', so-called because the functions measured by these tests are believed to be resistant to brain disease, and 'Don't Hold tests' which are more vulnerable. The 'Hold tests' involve the use of knowledge which has been acquired in the past, like vocabulary, information and verbal knowledge generally while the 'Don't

71

Hold tests' require speed or the acquisition of new knowledge or perception of new relations like digit symbol or the similarities test. In theory, a deterioration index derived from the tests might be expected to correspond with the progression and severity of a dementing process but in practice there is often insufficient definition from patients with functional psychiatric disorders.

The WAIS, as will also be seen in another section, has been subject to widespread criticism. Some of this has been technical and is to do with problems of standardizations. Age, cultural and social factors and secular change in norms are some of the points of criticism. Also the reliability of the individual sub-tests is thought suspect, especially in the detection of the more subtle changes. Yet, for all this, the WAIS is still widely used and is considered adequate for everyday use with demented patients.

The Halstead–Reitan Test Battery (HRTB)

Halstead first published his results in 1947 and Reitan extended the test battery in 1951 to measure a broad range of abilities. It consists of a number of independent tests but the composition of the battery can vary from laboratory to laboratory. The aim of the battery is not only to detect brain damage but to indicate whether this is likely to be focal or diffuse, lateralized to the right or left hemisphere, and whether acute, progressive or relatively static. So far, however, the battery has been used mainly for comparison between different categories of brain-damaged patients or between brain-damaged subjects and healthy controls.

The following account of the battery, which includes the WAIS and incorporates the tests described below, is based on the review by Golden *et al.* (1981). It is given in some detail as the HRTB is not in regular use in this country.

Halstead's category test

This consists of groups of pictures displayed on a screen, in response to which the subject must press one of four levers. There are certain unifying concepts which the patient must discover by trial and error. It is thus a relatively complex concept formation test which requires the subject to note similarities and differences, to set up hypotheses and to test and modify them. It is a measure of conceptual and problem-solving capacities and it is claimed to be 90% effective in distinguishing between brain-damaged and normal individuals.

Speech-sounds perception test

This consists of a series of tape-recorded nonsense words which the subject must identify by selection from printed alternatives. A poor performance is thought to indicate left temporal lobe dysfunction.

The seashore rhythm test

This requires the subject to differentiate between several pairs of rhythmic beats, assessing alertness, ability for sustained attention, and ability to perceive differing rhythm sequences. Deficits are thought to be due to right temporal lobe involvement.

Tactual performance test

This test requires the subject to fit blocks into their spaces on a board while blindfolded, and later to draw the board from memory. It requires tactile form discrimination, manual dexterity and co-ordination and the visualiza tion of spatial configurations. The skills required, there being no visual cues, are kinaesthetic/proprioceptive and the performance with either hand reflects the status of the contralateral hemisphere.

Trail-making test

This consists of 25 circles distributed over a sheet of paper. In the first part (Test A) the circles are numbered, and the subject must draw a line connecting them in numerical sequence as quickly as possible. In the second part (Part B) the circles contain both numbers and letters and the subject must alternate between numbers and letters as he proceeds in ascending sequence. The score is the time taken over the task. Errors must be corrected and are thus incorporated in the time score.

Performance on the test requires spatial analysis, motor control, ability to shift attention between alternatives, alertness, concentration and number and letter sense. Test A is a general measure of visuospatial scanning ability and motor and sequencing skills. It reflects right hemisphere integrity. Test B involves language symbol manipulation and is a measure of left hemisphere intactness. Therefore if one part remains intact a lateralized injury may be present. It is also claimed that Test B might be a sensitive indicator of brain damage in general.

Reitan–Klove sensory-perceptual examination

This measures both basic (e.g. finger agnosia) and more complex (e.g. astereognosis) sensory and perceptual processes and involves the use of touch in random sequence. The presence of lateralized deficits is thought to be a reliable indicator of brain dysfunction in the absence of peripheral disorders.

Reitan–Indiana aphasia examination

This contains items for testing ability to name objects, spell, identify single numbers and letters, read, write, calculate, name body parts and distinguish right from left. It is considered a reliable indicator of left hemisphere dysfunction.

Administration of the Halstead-Reitan Test Battery leads to the calculation of the Impairment Index which is a summary score representing perform- ance on the tests in the battery most sensitive to brain dysfunction in general. Anywhere from seven to twelve tests, depending on the number scored in the laboratory, may be included and the Impairment Index is calculated as follows:

$$\text{Impairment Index (II)} = \frac{\text{Number of tests in brain-damaged range}}{\text{Total number of tests}}$$

An index score greater than 0.4 is generally thought to be indicative of brain damage. Type, severity and chronicity of an injury are also thought to be reflected on the II. Fast-growing, destructive tumours cause the greatest II and slow-growing, non-destructive lesions cause less severe impairment. In general, II is believed to be lower in older lesions and with an acute injury the II will be high initially and decrease with time. In dementia the II is often 1.0, reflecting a generalized deterioration of brain function including those functions thought to be resistant to most brain damage (e.g. vocabulary).

In vascular disease, localized deficit may reflect the artery affected. If the left middle cerebral artery is involved, extensive verbal deficits may be expected; right middle cerebral lesions lead to severe spatial problems (e.g. with block design and drawings).

Though the interpretations of the findings of the battery appear to be attractively neat, all the criticisms made in the preamble to this chapter are as applicable to the Halstead–Reitan Test Battery as for other tests.

Wechsler Memory Scale (WMS)

This consists of seven sub-tests which attempt to measure several aspects of memory function. The raw score can be changed into a Memory Quotient which can be compared with the Intelligence Quotient.

The sub-tests consist of questions on *personal and current information, immediate orientation, mental control* (e.g. counting backwards from 20 to 1, repeating the alphabet), *logical memory, digit span, visual reproduction* (drawing geometrical figures from immediate memory) and *paired-associate learning.*

The WMS finds its widest use in enabling impaired memory function to be seen in the context of other cognitive dysfunction. It has its drawbacks in that the components of the impaired memory process are not reflected to any great extent in the test. There is also no measure of retention apart from the immediate. As Albert (1981) has pointed out, its most serious shortcoming is thought to be the confounding of perceptual and constructional skills with non-verbal memory. When evaluating visuospatial skills the ability to correctly perceive a stimulus should be assessed separately, it is said, from the ability to reproduce it so that perceptual impairment can be differentiated from constructional ones.

Rey–Osterrieth test

In this test the patient copies a single, complex geometrical design and then reproduces it from memory some time later. The patient copies the figure out so that artistic limitation, as well as disordered spatial perception, can be noted. The recall drawing is 40 minutes later and is a function of visual memory. It will be seen that it is a test which complements any that may be used for verbal memory. The test scores are intact in cases with dominant temporal lobe damage but are affected in lesions of the non-dominant temporal lobe.

The modified Kendrick battery

The original version of the Kendrick battery proved to be too stressful for many elderly patients. It consisted of two parts: the *synonym learning test* (SLT), which is a measure of short-term verbal memory, and the *digit copying test* (DCT) which is a measure of speed of simple information processing.

In the modified battery the SLT has been replaced by a test of visual short-term memory, the *object learning test* (OLT). This requires subjects to look at line drawings of familiar objects for a brief period, and then to recall as many as possible. The DCT from the original battery is retained with modification and larger digits.

The revised battery has been investigated with respect to its reliability and validity and norms now exist for normal, depressed and dementing subjects over 55 years of age. It is claimed it discriminates well between demented and non-dementing psychiatric patients and that the two tests are sensitive to cognitive change within individuals over time (Gibson *et al.*, 1980).

PSYCHOMETRY IN NORMAL OLD AGE

In evaluating an elderly person who presents with changes in cognitive functioning, the first task is to differentiate changes related to normal ageing from those due to pathology.

Age-appropriate norms based on a systematic comparison between elderly normal and pathological populations do not exist for most behavioural tests of brain damage (Albert, 1981). Most neuropsychological tests in use are based on the performance of young and middle-aged adults and since certain cognitive functions (e.g. memory) clearly change with age, norms relating to such abilities may not be applicable to the aged. Some cognitive functions appear to be maintained with age (e.g. digit span forward), however, and young adult norms may well be appropriate in many instances.

Albert takes up the question of valid norms further in relation to some of the commoner tests used in investigating the aged patient. Most age-connected norms have been developed from cross-sectional studies and as such may only be cohort-specific. Not only are the educational attainment and health status of these groups likely to differ but the language patterns and problem-solving styles of successive generations may have changed as well. This may mean that 1960 norms need to be adjusted to today's elderly population (Albert, 1981). Taking up the recent criticism of the norms for older persons regarding WAIS and the HRTB, Albert reports that the problems with WAIS have been attributed to the fact that while younger individuals' IQ norms are derived from a nationwide sample, subjects over 65 have to make do with norms obtained from smaller, more geographically limited groups. Hence the criticism of unrepresentative sampling. Another is that there has been inadequate correction for changes in performance IQ over time.

As for the HRTB, the consequence of inadequate normative data is that 'cut-off' scores for brain damage have to be obtained from younger patients. A result of this compromise has been that as many as 90% of elderly subjects, including one series of especially 'well-functioning, active and involved' elderly citizens, have had scores in the abnormal range of the trail-making test and tactual performance test of the HRTB. Perhaps the greatest criticism of psychological test results in clinical practice has been the number of false-positives they throw up, and this problem seems compounded in the elderly patient.

Quite apart from cognitive functioning *per se* other factors that need to be kept in mind when elderly patients are being assessed are differences in motivation, expectation of performance, easy fatiguability and motor and sensory changes.

It is also becoming clear, as Albert has further pointed out, that the general state of health of elderly subjects must be kept in mind. It is thought that systemic diseases such as diabetes, lung disease, heart disease and hypertension can all affect cognitive function, with evidence being presented that mildly hypertensive patients have perceptual and psychomotor impairments that are reduced by anti-hypertensive medication. The areas of investigation are usually

(1) attention;
(2) language;
(3) memory;
(4) abstraction;
(5) cognitive flexibility;
(6) visuospatial ability.

It is clear that attention, upon which all cognitive performance rests, must be evaluated at the outset. A detailed examination would include both auditory (e.g. digit span) and well as visual attention (e.g. numbers being crossed out) as there can be selective impairment.

Tests on language include an evaluation of comprehension, reading, repetition, writing and naming. Aspects of memory are tested in the manner discussed in the previous section with both verbal and non-verbal memory being submitted to examination. The simplest method of evaluating abstraction is by proverb interpretation. More detailed assessment is via the Wisconsin card sorting test, in which geometrical figures in various shapes and colours are give to be sorted out by the patient. He is required to sort colour, form and number following a stimulus and shift from one to another. Thus both the ability to categorize as well as to change a cognitive frame of reference – thought to be elements of frontal lobe function – are needed.

One of the difficulties in evaluating current cognitive performance is that the psychologist is usually unaware of the previous level of functioning of the patient. The vocabulary sub-test of the WAIS, which belongs to the

'Hold' category of tests, is often said to be a quick estimate of premorbid ability. This is generally true if cognitive status is not seriously impaired but may not be applicable to cases of dementia where more serious forms of cognitive impairment are expected. Occupation, educational and social information, gathered in the course of history taking, may often prove the most satisfactory guide to premorbid cognitive status.

In the case of many tests it is futile to expect exact or accurate localization. The idea of a seat of the soul is not given much credence in modern psychology. Most tests require many different abilities (e.g. psychomotor, visuospatial, memory) to complete successfully. Their usefulness is in drawing attention to dysfunction and in the relatively unspecific localization of verbal or non-verbal deficit.

Memory is a far more complex function than is suggested by the relatively simple nature of the tests used. A straightforward failure to recall an answer, for instance, might well be just that or a failure of transfer between, or retrieval from, any of the number of memory stores that are postulated to exist. The underlying pathology might be very different even when overt disorder is the same. The case for detailed examination of any symptom of cognitive dysfunction must be a strong one.

As with measurements of IQ, most measures of memory functioning must depend ultimately on the ability and willingness of the patient to respond. These include mood, personality and certain other factors which have been mentioned before.

PSYCHOMETRY IN DEMENTIA

Perez (1980), among others, believes the evaluation of the behavioural changes associated with dementia has been accomplished by way of neuropsychological test batteries which, unfortunately, suffer from a number of methodological as well as practical problems. Some of these have been dealt with in the foregoing paragraphs in a general consideration of neuropsychological assessment and are worth re-stating with respect to dementia. They include:

(1) imprecise or non-specific measures which do not differentiate kinds of dysfunction or reflect structural pathology;
(2) insensitive tests which do not detect instances of disability or accurately reflect the degree of impairment;
(3) procedures which do not adequately control for differences in motivational states between individuals;
(4) test environments which promote extraneous patient–clinician interactions that subsequently bias test results;
(5) test material which is prejudiced, biased or irrelevant to the problem being diagnosed, i.e. material that is dependent on the patient's particular social and educational background (Perez, 1980).

Blackburn (1979) has considered the questions that present themselves to a psychologist when confronted with a demented patient to be examined and followed up, with treatment, over a period of time.

(1) What should be the content of the tests?
(2) At what level should the tests be pitched?
(3) Should they be nomothetic or idiographic?
(4) How often and where should patients be tested?

It is generally agreed that the tests must tap attention, concentration and orientation, language, memory, abstract thought, cognitive flexibility, the agnosias and apraxias.

The length of time over which a demented patient can be tested corresponds to the time the patient can be satisfactorily assessed clinically, i.e. 30–45 minutes.

Comprehensive test batteries are used with sacrifice of sensitivity. For instance, as Blackburn (1979) has noted from a study of demented patients, with a more detailed testing of different aspects of memory it would have been possible to detect diminution in intellectual function in patients at an early stage of their illness. Similarly, a more flexible approach to testing is likely to be more fruitful because it might be geared to suit the variability in level of functioning which is found in Alzheimer's disease. An *idiographic* approach would concentrate on each individual's dysfunction, establish his base line level and then study the progression of the disease or response to treatment. The part *nomothetic* approach Blackburn adopted, with sub-tests borrowed from several sources, proved to be 'fairly useless' for both well-preserved and severely deteriorated patients.

Even demented patients get used to the practice effects of tests which should not therefore be repeated at too frequent intervals. This also saves psychologists' time. However, in one of her more surprising conclusions Blackburn has said the best behavioural rating is often made by nurses. With training, discussion and feedback, nurses seemed to produce ratings which were valid, reliable and useful. The most convenient place of testing is usually a psychologist's office or, for behavioural ratings, a hospital ward. But patients do best in their homes, which is the most familiar ground for them. A compromise place of testing would be a research ward where patients were allowed to settle for at least 2 weeks before assessment.

Blackburn concludes that it is possible to obtain valid and sensitive measures by combining daily behavioural rating with formal assessment. The latter should preferably combine a wide enough approach (covering several areas of dysfunction) with detailed flexible testing of the main dysfunction, i.e. of memory, where each individual's limit can be tested.

In concluding this section it must be said that clinicians, always aware of the rather amorphous nature of their data, have had attitudes ranging from sheer disbelief to blind faith in psychologists' ability to mesmerise them with numbers. The most useful position to hold, in an attitude of informed scepticism, is probably somewhere in the middle between these two.

We shall leave the last word to a psychologist, Marcer (1979):

> For a few psychologists the search for the right Wechsler sub-test combination still goes on, rather like the mediaeval alchemists' search for the philosopher's stone, and with as little likelihood of ultimate success. Occasionally, reports of new indices which seem to approach

useful levels of discrimination do appear . . . but these either lack the crucial confirmation by cross-validation or break down when attempts at cross-validation are made.

'Pseudo-dementia'

It has been put about that the intellectual dysfunction in this intriguing condition is a manifestation of lowered motivation, preoccupation with the affective state or a learned disability (Miller, 1977). These theories view the neuropsychological dysfunction as a by-product of the psychiatric disturbance. It is equally possible, of course, that the cognitive abnormalities reflect a neurochemical disturbance that produces specific impairment in brain function via the limbic system.

Even though pseudo-dementia patients fail many of the same tests on which dementia patients perform poorly (e.g. memory) it has been argued that their variability of performance from test to test best distinguishes them from patients with progressive disease (Wells, 1979).

There may well be a gradient of mental impairment from depression to dementia with normality proceeding through uncomplicated affective disorder to cognitive impairment. Caine (1981) has stated that pseudo-dementia patients show selective disorders of arousal, mental processing speed, spontaneous elaboration and analysis of detail. Memory disturbance was present in his patients, but it was thought to be secondary to an attentional dysfunction. Problems with naming, writing and calculation were minimal. The pattern of intellectual impairment seen in 'pseudo-dementia' is therefore a 'subcortical' one, a concept discussed in Chapter 3.

Alzheimer's disease

The presentation of Alzheimer's disease can vary but memory loss is most often the earliest feature. Both short-term and remote memory may be affected. The other early testable clinical features are difficulties with abstract reasoning, concept formation and general cognitive flexibility.

Though Alzheimer's disease is a progressive, diffuse disorder affecting both hemispheres it is not unusual, as we shall note later, to find obvious cognitive impairment stemming from one or the other hemisphere. Thus difficulties with speech and other symbolic function may be affected in the absence of visuospatial disturbance and vice-versa. Memory difficulties are less easy to trace to one hemisphere in practice. A particularly sinister phenomenon is expressive language deficit, which is known to be related to mortality in the year after testing.

Recent studies have reported on the correlation between the extent of the neuropathological features of Alzheimer's disease, such as neurofibrillary tangles and senile plaques and cognitive impairment. Another finding has been that neurofibrillary tangles and granulovacuolar changes are most obvious in the hippocampus-limbic system which seems to subserve certain types of memory function (Tomlinson et al., 1970; Terry and Wisniewski, 1973).

Conventional wisdom has had it that while multi-infarct or vascular dementia seemed to progress by fits and starts in a 'step-wise' fashion, Alzheimer's disease ran a smoother, progressive course. In psychometric terms this is, in fact, not always so, and often after a period of relative stability or a gradual fall in performance on tests, an abrupt drop may occur in the few months or the year before death from Alzheimer's disease.

The more specific psychometric impairments in Alzheimer's disease are considered in the next section, when they are contrasted with those of vascular dementia.

Multi-infarct or vascular dementia

General intellectual impairment is believed to become evident when multi-infarct disease leads to the destruction of more that 50 ml of brain tissue.

Several studies (e.g. Perez *et al.*, 1975, 1976) have attempted to discriminate between patients with Alzheimer's disease and multi-infarct dementia on the basis of cognitive test scores. Alzheimer disease patients seemed to be significantly impaired on the performance scale of the WAIS. Perez *et al.* (1975) found the Alzheimer disease group performing significantly and consistently lower on all intellectual measures. A discriminant function analysis classified 74% of the patients correctly using the individual WAIS scores. The discrimination was more easily made when tasks measuring visual motor co-ordination and abstract reasoning were included in the analysis. The data also seemed to suggest that the multi-infarct group was less homogeneous than the Alzheimer disease group, as might have been predicted from the patchy nature of the disease process in the former. The degree and pattern of intellectual deficit, as might also have been expected, varied with each multi-infarct dementia patient depending on the site, location, extent and number of cerebral infarctions.

Different patterns of memory performance using the Wechsler Memory Scale (WMS) were found by Perez *et al.* (1975) in patients with Alzheimer's disease and multi-infarct dementia. Statistically it could be revealed that the Alzheimer disease group again performed significantly and consistently poorly on all memory measures. A discriminant function analysis classified 100% of the patients correctly using their individual WMS score. The discrimination was primarily based on the memory quotient (MQ) score and the individual performance on the paired associate sub-test, which studies the ability to learn and remember new verbal information, which is more seriously affected in Alzheimer's disease.

In general, therefore, it seems that in Alzheimer's disease the dementing disorder affects memory significantly more than other cognitive abilities though virtually all aspects of higher function can be affected in the disease.

Perez *et al.* (1978) proposed the rather elegantly simple hypothesis that since multi-infarct dementia was more likely to be due to discrete focal lesions of one cerebral hemisphere, a test investigating motor function disturbance of the two hands was more likely to show a right–left-hand difference in this disease than in Alzheimer's disease, which can be presumed to involve diffuse general lesions of both cerebral hemispheres. The test used was the finger-tapping test which compares the fine finger motor dexterity of the preferred hand to the non-preferred, and is highly sensitive to unilateral cerebral disease with decrements on the opposite side. They found the hypothesis could be gratifyingly upheld at cost only to Popperian ideas about science.

Huntington's chorea

When suspected, it is possible that the chorea may not be evident, and in view of the peculiarly distressing effects of the disease there is an even greater than usual urgency for early diagnosis. Memory deficits may be an early and prominent feature, but so might they be in early Alzheimer's disease. The distinction may be made by subjecting the patient to confrontation naming. This is impaired in Alzheimer's disease but may be preserved in Huntington's chorea.

The EEG, cerebral blood flow and computerized tomographic correlates of impaired cognitive function are considered in turn in each of the next three chapters.

SUMMARY

(1) The purpose of psychometry in dementia is to assess the cognitive and behavioural changes found or suspected on clinical examination in quantitative terms.

(2) Psychometry is important in three areas: (a) in quantifying and establishing a baseline for intellectual, memory and other cognitive functions; (b) in testing and measuring areas of specific dysfunction in the patient's behaviour so as to assist in a differential diagnosis; (c) in helping plan management and rehabilitation.

(3) Psychometric tests can only be interpreted in conjunction with all other clinical information. There is no one psychometric test valid for all cases showing brain damage, and misleading information may be obtained in patients whose dysfunction is less than clear-cut.

(4) The larger the number of functions sampled by the test, the greater will be its usefulness as a general screening device, though a price will then have to be paid in a sacrifice of sensitivity in detecting minor degrees of dysfunction in more restricted areas of cognitive activity.

(5) Neuropsychological tests are based on the assumption that verbal and symbolic activity in general is a function of parts of the dominant hemisphere and visuospatial activity is dependent on the integrity of parts of the non-dominant hemisphere.

(6) The Wechsler Adult Intelligence Scale (WAIS) is made up of six tests of verbal intellectual function and five tests of performance intelligence. The six tests measuring verbal IQ are information, comprehension, arithmetic, similarities, digit span and vocabulary sub-tests.

The five tests measuring performance IQ include digit symbol, picture completeness, block design, picture arrangement and object assembly sub-tests.

(7) The independent tests in the Halstead–Reitan Test Battery (HRTB) include the WAIS and the following:

(a)	Halstead's category test	– Conceptual skills and problem solving.
(b)	Speech-sounds perception test	– Left temporal lobe function.
(c)	Seashore rhythm test	– Right temporal lobe function.
(d)	Tactual performance test	– Status of contralateral hemisphere.
(e)	Trail making test:	
	Test A	– Right hemisphere integrity;
	Test B	– Left hemisphere integrity.
(f)	Reitan–Klove sensory perceptual examination	– Basic (e.g. finger agnosia) and more complex (e.g. astereognosis) sensory and perceptual processes.
(g)	Reitan–Indiana aphasia examination	– Left hemisphere function.

(8) The Wechsler Memory Scale (WMS) has the following sub-tests:
  (a) Personal and current information.
  (b) Immediate orientation.
  (c) Mental control.
  (d) Logical memory.
  (e) Digit span forwards and backwards.
  (f) Visual reproduction.
  (g) Paired-associate learning.

(9) The Rey–Osterrieth test examines performance or visuo-spatial memory function.

(10) The Kendrick battery includes the synonym learning test (SLT) for short-term verbal memory *or* the object learning test (OLT) for short-term visual memory *and* the digit copying test (DCT) for simple information processing.

(11) The Wisconsin card sorting test examines frontal lobe function.

(12) In testing elderly patients, care should be taken to see that appropriate norms for cognitive function are used. These may differ markedly from young adult norms.

(13) In assessing cognitive function in the elderly it is important to bear in mind the changes that might be due to motivation, caution, lowered expectations, fatiguability, motor, sensory and reflex changes and any history of systemic disease and drug intake.

(14) It is recommended that six areas of investigation be carried out: attention, language, memory, abstraction, cognitive flexibility and visuospatial ability.

(15) It is possible to obtain valid and sensitive results by combining daily behavioural ratings with formal assessment.

(16) There may be a gradient of impairment from depression to dementia ranging from normality through uncomplicated affective disorder to cognitive impairment. Patients with 'pseudo-dementia' seem to show a high variability of performance.

(17) Both short-term and remote memory impairment are found in Alzheimer's disease, and memory loss is very often the earliest presenting symptom. Expressive language deficits appear to correlate with mortality within a year.

(18) In multi-infarct dementia (vascular dementia) destruction of more than 50 ml of brain tissue seems to lead to general cognitive impairment.

(19) Alzheimer disease patients, when compared to comparable patients with multi-infarct or vascular dementia, perform significantly and consistently lower on all intellectual measures.

(20) The degree and pattern of intellectual deficit varies with each multi-infarct dementia patient and depends on the site, location, extent and number of cerebral infarctions.

(21) Huntington's chorea may present with disordered short-term and remote memory disturbance as the only neuropsychological deficit. It may be possible to distinguish this from Alzheimer's disease by considering language function, especially confrontation naming of objects, which is affected in Alzheimer' disease and preserved in Huntington's chorea.

Further reading

(A full list of references is given at the end of the book)

Albert, M.S. (1981). Geriatric neuropsychology. *J. Consult. Clin. Psychol.*, **49** (6), 835-850
Lishman, W.A. (1978). *Organic Psychiatry*. (London: Blackwell Scientific Publications)

5
The electroencephalogram in dementia

For he maketh the storm to cease: so that the waves thereof are still.
Then they are glad, because they are at rest: and so he bringeth them   into the heaven where they would be.

Book of Common Prayer, 1662

The electroencephalogram (EEG) as an instrument for the study of brain function and dysfunction has the advantage of being non-invasive and cheap, and causing little discomfort or danger. Unlike, say, cerebral biopsy, the standard procedure for recording an EEG does not raise ethical questions, and serial studies for the purposes of mapping the course of an illness as well as normal variation are possible. It also has the advantage of having a body of knowledge going back some 50 years. Berger (1932), for instance, had already described the slowing of the waking, resting EEG in senile dementia patients as compared to healthy old persons. As will be seen shortly, this finding is the starting point even today in the EEG evaluation of the demented patient.

With the advent of computerized tomography (CT) in the 1970s and the rush into routine and indiscriminate head scanning, the role of traditional neurological investigatory tools has come to be questioned. However, Rosenberg *et al.* (1982), after studying 136 patients without focal neurological features by EEG and CT found the likelihood of finding lesions on CT increased with appearance of signs of focal EEG dysfunction, and thought the older and cheaper investigation served as a useful screen.

With the possibility of pharmacological therapy in at least some cases of dementia increasingly likely, therapeutic monitoring and control of optimal dosages of drugs may also be feasible with regular EEG recordings.

This chapter on aspects of the EEG in dementia begins with an outline of the possible limits to normal variation, especially in relation to age. Where abnormality passes definitely into pathology is, of course, as moot with the EEG as with many other physiological measurements. Be that as it may, we then move on to consider the EEG correlates of the dementia syndrome. A natural step from there is to go on to discuss EEG changes in specific disorders leading to dementia. Finally, the intriguing possibility that there might exist a generalized physiological dysfunction of the body in dementia is taken up briefly in a consideration of EEG changes in relation to blood pressure, metabolic rate and sleep.

SOME NORMAL VARIATIONS

The EEG being a measure of brain function it seems only natural to expect changes in it with alterations in the physiological status of individuals. Changes in the EEG in one of those parameters – normal old age – have been noted by several authors (e.g. Obrist and Busse, 1965; Muller, 1978).

Consistent findings with normal old age seem to include the following:

(1) slowing of background (alpha) rhythm frequencies;
(2) changes in fast frequency activity (normally increases in the theta range);
(3) the appearance of slow waves, especially in the temporal regions and more commonly in the left hemisphere;
(4) decrease of reactivity of the EEG to hyperventilation and to stimulation.

The dominant frequency of the EEG slows with age but usually remains within the alpha range in normal old age.

Otomo (1966), studying normal subjects, found the distribution shown in Table 5.1.

Table 5.1 Distribution of alpha frequency in normal old age (after Otomo, 1966)

Decade	Alpha frequencies (cps)
7th	9.67±1.04[*]
8th	9.50±1.02[*] [**]
9th	9.07±1.50[**]

[*] Statistically significant at 5% level
[**] Statistically significant at 1% level

Otomo (1966) further studied normal subjects, non-neurological patients and neurological patients. His results are shown in Table 5.2.

Table 5.2 Distribution of alpha frequencies amongst three groups (after Otomo, 1966)

Subjects	Alpha frequency (cps)
Normal	9.47±1.73[*]
Non-neurological patients	9.01±1.52
Neurological patients	8.65±1.64[*]

[*] Significant at 5% level

In addition to significant slowing of alpha rhythms, the neurological patients also had more abnormality of slow wave activity. Otomo also considered the distribution curve of the 9th decade of the normals and, finding it similar to that of the neurological patients, was led to wonder if the 9th decade might represent a physiologically critical point.

Some years before this, Obrist (1954) had noted that more normal old people than young have frequencies in the theta range, and Busse *et al.* (1956) had remarked that localized temporal slow wave activity was common in normal old age.

A physiological variable which has EEG correlates in both sickness and health is sleep. The EEG findings in the sleep of demented patients are considered later in this chapter but Obrist (1978a) has noted that among the more sensitive age-related variables are changes in all-night EEG sleep patterns during normal ageing. Sleep patterns become fragmented, so that awakenings are longer and more frequent than in young adults. This is associated with a marked reduction in stage 4 sleep (high-voltage delta waves) and a moderate decrease in the time occupied by dream or rapid eye movement (REM) sleep. In addition, there is a significant decline in the number of 12–14 cps spindle bursts which are replaced by lower-frequency spindle-like rhythms. The decrease in REM sleep is of particular interest because it is highly correlated with impairment on intelligence and memory tests. Furthermore, the decline in REM sleep is consistent with age-related pathological changes observed in the *locus coeruleus*, a brain stem structure believed to modulate REM activity, possibly through cholinergic mechanisms. The significance of this to dementia is considered later.

Some authors (e.g. Maggs and Turton, 1956) have commented that elevated blood pressure may be associated with a relatively high incidence of normal EEG tracings in aged psychiatric patients, although in normal subjects such a correlation was not observed (Obrist *et al.*, 1961). Otomo (1966) also found no difference in the incidence of abnormal EEG between normotensive and hypertensive groups of patients. The significance of the relationship of the EEG to blood pressure is also taken up in a later section of this chapter.

ALZHEIMER'S DISEASE

The central EEG feature in Alzheimer's disease appears to be progressive diffuse slowing followed by disorganization of the rhythm, i.e. it becomes random in occurrence and irregular in frequency. The slowing of the alpha activity may go below the 7 cps which can also be observed in healthy old age (Muller, 1978). Roberts *et al.* (1976) have reviewed several studies which have shown that with increasing degrees of intellectual impairment, slow dominant frequencies become even more common. The correlation with decline of mental function is quite strong and Muller (1978) estimates it may be up to 0.8.

There is also said to be significant correlation between the number of senile plaques and slowing of the alpha rhythm (Diesenhammer and Jellinger, 1974).

Roberts *et al.* (1976) also remark that dominant delta (slow wave) activity was found only in those with moderate or severe intellectual deficit. The relatively late manifestation of EEG features is also remarked on by Harner (1975), who states that over the course of 1 or more years progressive diffuse slowing and loss of fast activity occur but lag behind clinical symptoms until the last stages when even paroxysmal or 'triphasic' (spike and slow wave) activity may be seen. Occasionally, the rapid slowing of the alpha rhythm in dementia helps it to be distinguished from uncomplicated ageing in serial EEG tracings.

Although the slow activity in Alzheimer's disease is usually disorganized, some patients with severe dementia, however, show rhythmic bursts of bilaterally synchronous delta waves that are maximal over the frontal and temporal regions. Not very surprisingly, it has been suggested that the severity of EEG slowing in Alzheimer's disease is related to the rapidity of the dementing process.

EEG slowing also seems to distinguish between functional and organic patients, and claims have been made for its value in predicting survival. Apparently, only a few patients with diffusely slow tracings survive beyond 5 years, while most of those with normal EEG tracings do so. A study bearing upon this is tabulated in Table 5.3.

The presence of fast activity in normal old age, on the other hand, can be regarded as a favourable sign for intellectual function and tends to disappear with senile deterioration. Muller (1978) has speculated that sharp and fast activity might be expressions of a neurobiological effort to counteract decreasing brain functions, perhaps in terms of a more active search for structure.

Table 5.3 EEG findings related to diagnosis and prognosis in 90 aged psychiatric patients (after Obrist, 1978a).

	No. of patients by diagnosis		No. of patients by outcome after 1 year	
EEG finding	Functional disorder (n=45)	Organic dementia (n=45)	Discharged or convalescent (n=45)	Hospitalized or dead (n=45)
Normal tracing	28	4	23	9
Diffuse slow waves*	2	30	9	23
Slow alpha rhythm*	8	16	10	14
Focal slow activity*	8	7	8	7

* These functions may be found together

OTHER DEMENTIAS

Once the EEG correlates of the clinical syndrome of dementia are established, the tracings can be examined further for clues as to aetiological processes other than Alzheimer's disease. A summary of findings described in the text is given in Table 5.4.

Harner (1975) has noted that most treatable causes of dementias are associated with prominent EEG abnormalities, while primary or 'degenerative' causes such as Alzheimer' disease, which are for the most part untreatable, show few EEG abnormalities in the early stages of development unless the rate of progression is rapid.

Striano *et al.* (1981) note that the EEG tracings observed in multi-infarct or vascular dementias are characterized by lack of severe abnormality in the background activity, by the rarity of bursts of delta wave activity, by good reactivity (i.e. response to hyperventilation and stimulation) and by the high incidence of focal abnormalities. The last are more often localized to or prevalent on the right side, particularly in the parieto-temporal areas. Speculating as to the significance of this, they feel this finding supports the view that the right hemisphere's predominant function is in processing visuospatial performance, a function which needs relatively large cortical areas in contrast to language function which is dependent on extremely specialized 'centres'. Global deterioration of mental function is therefore likely to be associated with lesions of the non-dominant hemisphere with impairment of visuospatial functions, whereas dominant hemisphere lesions result in more specific neurological disturbances in the clinical picture.

In a series of 32 cerebrovascular, 40 Alzheimer disease and 25 mixed cases of dementia, Constantinidis *et al.* (1969) observed three times more alpha rhythm (7–8 cps) in patients with vascular lesions and fives times more theta and delta foci. Patients with Alzheimer's disease, on the other hand, had a significantly higher incidence of diffuse delta activity.

However, slow wave activity in sites other than the temporal lobe is noted to be considerably more common in dementia of vascular origin than in Alzheimer's disease. Roberts *et al.* (1976), in their series comparing vascular with non-vascular dements with CT and EEG, found reasonable correlation between physical signs, the presence of visible infarct and the site of slow wave activity. Obrist (1978a) confirms that in dementia due to cerebrovascular disease, background rhythms, though slow, are generally well preserved and there is a higher incidence of focal (as opposed to diffuse) slow activity.

In this connection it has to be borne in mind that confusion can arise when features such as language disturbance, focal weakness or seizure occur in the course of a degenerative disorder. These clinical findings may be mirrored in the EEG as focal slow wave or focal irritative activity (sharp waves, spikes) (Harner, 1975).

The advent of computerized tomography (CT) has enabled anatomical lesions to be compared with the physiological dysfunction traced by the EEG. Roberts *et al.* (1976), while noting earlier findings that in non-vascular dementia the degree of EEG abnormality and degree of ventricular dilation could be related to the severity of mental impairment, were unable to confirm a correlation between ventricular size detectable on CT and EEG features. They conclude that since EEG changes reflect disordered cortical function rather than loss of cerebral substance any lack of relationship should not be surprising.

As Harner (1975) has remarked, the usefulness of EEG evaluation in patients is dependent on the stage of development of symptoms. In the early stages, a normal EEG constitutes good evidence against metabolic, toxic, focal or infectious causes. In the later stages the presence of diffuse slowing helps in the distinction between organic causes of dementia and those of functional origin.

Hyponatraemia, hypothyroidism, hypercalcaemia, pernicious anaemia, uraemia, hepatic encephalopathy and pulmonary insufficiency are characterized by diffuse slow activity, which usually antedates the onset of mental symptoms and correlates with the degree of impairment (Harner, 1975). In addition, irritative features are common in anoxia and disorders of electrolyte metabolism. Triphasic waves appear in 20% of patients with uraemic and hepatic encephalopathy, and focal slow wave activity may also occur, presumably due to pre-existing areas of decreased resistance in the brain (Harner, 1975).

Muller (1978) analysed 24 cases of triphasic (sharp and slow wave dysfunction) on the EEG. His results were as shown in Table 5.4. The results appear to suggest that dementia, uncomplicated by systemic illness, can give rise to triphasic waves on the EEG. Muller (1978) suggests that the brain disorder imposed on systemic illness produces triphasic waves but their presence alone cannot suggest dementia.

Since the dementing syndrome represents the severe, late state of metabolic encephalopathy Harner (1975) believes the EEG will be abnormal in virtually every case, and therefore might be a very useful screening procedure. However, he is well aware that confusion can arise with hypothermia, hypothyroidism and vitamin B_{12} deficiency, each of which can produce gradual slowing of alpha activity indistinguishable from the slowing that can occur as part of the normal ageing process or in the early stages of Alzheimer's disease.

He also believes that the EEG used in conjunction with ultrasound estimations of brain mass is an excellent screening procedure for the detection of localized brain lesions, especially those that have grown sufficiently large to produce symptoms of dementia. Rapidly growing primary tumours and metastatic lesions are said to be most easily detected but parasagittal and basal meningiomas are also evident by the time they have grown large enough to produce dementia. This combined procedure also helps eliminate false positives in the diagnosis of subdural haematomata (SDH). In their experience the EEG shows some abnormality in 90% of cases of SDH and is of lateralizing value in about 80%.

On the other hand, in Pick's disease, even in the advanced stages, the EEG is remarkable for its normality (Johannesson et al., 1977). The EEG pattern in Creutzfeldt-Jakob disease is invariably described as characteristic at least in the later stages, and consists of periodic outbursts of spike and slow wave activity occurring at regular intervals (Harner, 1975). Similar patterns may be observed in other degenerative conditions of the brain but confusion should not arise when the full clinical picture is taken into account.

The allegedly distinctive nature of the 'flat', low-voltage EEG in Huntington's chorea was once thought to hold considerable promise for the pre-symptomatic detection of this dreaded illness, but this interest has now waned.

Table 5.5 summarizes the EEG appearances in major causes of dementia.

Table 5.4   Causes of triphasic waves on EEG (after Muller, 1978)

Liver dysfunction	2
Other systemic disorders (pulmonary or abdominal infections)	7
Cerebrovascular disease (often with lateralization of triphasic wave)	6
Uncomplicated severe senile dementia – Alzheimer type	7
Unclear diagnosis	2

SOME PHYSIOLOGICAL CORRELATES OF THE EEG IN DEMENTIA

Blood pressure (BP)

Obrist *et al.* (1961) reported the incidence of diffuse slow activity (theta and delta) was inversely related to BP level in aged demented patients. Diminished cerebral blood flow (CBF) is a possible intermediary in this and, as Obrist (1978a) has observed, it requires the assumption that a moderately reduced blood pressure can adversely affect the cerebral circulation, a phenomenon that can only occur if blood flow autoregulation is impaired. This author's alternative explanation is that degenerative brain changes associated with slower EEG frequencies are responsible for lower BP, quite independently of any impaired haemodynamic influence on the EEG. The relationship between blood pressure and EEG tracings has not been observed in normal subjects.

Metabolic rate

In elderly patients with dementia Obrist *et al.* (1961) found significant correlation between EEG frequency and cerebral O_2-consumption, such that increased slow activity was associated with a reduced metabolic rate. On the other hand, they found no corresponding relationship in normal elderly subjects, which implies that the relationship depends on the existence of cerebral pathology. Such findings are difficult to interpret because it is not known if diminished blood flow is the cause of a lower metabolic rate, or if it merely represents an autoregulatory adjustment to the lesser metabolic demands of the tissue. In the demented patients above, cerebral arterio-venous O_2 differences were normal, indicating an absence of ischaemia at the time of study and suggesting that the blood flow reduction was secondary to lower metabolism. Obrist (1978a) believes that cerebral metabolism rather than blood flow is the primary variable affecting EEG frequency which is consistent with the higher correlation obtained with metabolic rate. This discussion is followed up further in Chapter 6.

Sleep

Among elderly patients with dementia, EEG sleep patterns undergo similar but more pronounced alterations than are observed in normal ageing (Obrist, 1978a). Feinberg *et al.* (1967) found longer and more numerous periods of wakefulness, greater reductions in stage 4 sleep and amount of spindle activity, and a striking decrease in rapid eye movement (REM) sleep. Again, Obrist (1978a) notes, this last variable was significantly correlated with impaired intellectual performance, as was the reduction in the number of spindles. These led Feinberg *et al.* (1967) to propose a common pathophysiology for the mechanism underlying sleep disturbance and cognition. Obrist (1978a) has also noted that in demented patients there is an additional tendency for sleep and waking patterns to become similar, in that both are dominated by irregular diffuse slow activity. As a further point of interest it is known that cholinergic mechanisms are involved in REM sleep, which may be induced with physostigmine and arecholine.

Table 5.5   A summary of EEG findings in dementia

With minimal or late EEG change	*With early EEG change*
Alzheimer or other 'primary illness degenerative'	*Multi-infarct dementia*
	1. Lacks severe abnormality of alpha rhythm in background activity.
Alzheimer's disease	2. High incidence of focal abnormality including slow wave activity.
1. EEG findings lag behind clinical features.	3. Bursts of delta activity and diffuse delta activity rare.
2. Progressive diffuse slowing of alpha rhythm.	4. Good reactivity present.
3. Slowing increases with severity of dementia.	*'Secondary' dementia – metabolic, toxic, infectious*
4. Delta slow waves in moderate/severe dementia – heralds poor prognosis.	1. Early EEG change.
5. Fast activity may be prognostically favourable.	2. Diffuse slow activity antedating onset of mental symptoms and correlating with impairment.
6. 'Triphasic' activity rare and terminal.	3. Irritative features common, especially in anoxia and electrolyte disturbance.
Pick's disease	4. 'Triphasic' waves, especially in uraemic and hepatic encephalopathy.
1. EEG may be normal even in advanced cases.	
Creutzfeldt–Jakob disease	
1. EEG changes follow clinical manifestations.	
2. In late stages – periodic bursts of spike and slow wave activity.	

SUMMARY

(1) The EEG is a cheap, non-invasive tool which causes little discomfort or danger to the patient and can be repeated serially. In patients with no focal features the EEG may be a useful screen to detect those likely to have abnormalities on CT. Also, changes in the EEG may come to be used to monitor effects of drugs used in dementia.

(2) Normal ageing produces changes on the EEG. These are slowing of the alpha rhythm, the appearance of slow waves, especially in the left temporal region, changes in fast frequency activity and a decrease of reactivity to hyperventilation and to stimulation. A critical decade for significant EEG changes in the elderly normal might be the 9th.

(3) The central EEG feature in Alzheimer's disease is a progressive

diffuse slowing followed by random and irregular disorganization of the rhythm.

The alpha rhythm may fall below 7 cps and is related to the number of senile plaques. Dominant delta (slow wave) activity is found in those with moderate/severe dementia. It is of poor prognostic import; few patients with these surviving for longer than 5 years.

The presence of fast activity may be favourable.

(4) Most treatable causes of dementia are associated with prominent, early EEG abnormalities while primary causes such as Alzheimer's disease show few EEG changes in the early stages.

In multi-infarct or vascular dementia there is lack of severe abnormality in the background alpha activity, diffuse delta activity is rare, there is good reactivity and a high incidence of focal abnormality.

Hyponatraemia, hypothyroidism, hypercalcaemia, pernicious anaemia, uraemia, hepatic encephalopathy and pulmonary insufficiency are characterized by diffuse slow activity which antedates onset of mental symptoms and correlates with degree of impairment.

Irritative features (spikes and sharp waves) are common in anoxia and disorders of electrolyte metabolism. Triphasic waves appear in 20% of cases of uraemic and hepatic encephalopathy. Used with ultrasound the EEG detects abnormality in the majority of cases of subdural haematoma leading to dementia.

In Pick's disease the EEG may be normal even in advanced clinical stages of illness.

In Creutzfeldt–Jakob disease the EEG shows a characteristic spike and wave activity in the later stages.

The flat voltage EEG of Huntington's chorea was once thought to hold promise in the pre-symptomatic detection of the illness but this is no longer held to be so.

(5) Diffuse EEG slow activity seems inversely related to blood pressure in aged demented patients. One explanation offered is that degenerative changes in the brain cause both the slowing of the EEG and the fall in blood pressure. Another is that autoregulation of cerebral blood flow is impaired.

Increased slow activity on the EEG is associated with reduced metabolic rate in demented patients. This may again be due to degenerative changes leading to lower metabolic demand.

Elderly demented patients have longer and more numerous periods of wakefulness, greater reduction in stage 4 sleep and spindle activity and diminished REM sleep. REM sleep reduction correlates with intellectual deterioration. A common pathophysiology underlying sleep disturbance and cognition has been proposed.

Further reading

(A full list of references is given at the end of the book)

Harner, R.N. (1975). EEG evaluation of the patient with dementia. In Benson, D.F. and Blumer, D. (eds). *Psychiatric Aspects of Neurological Disease.* (New York: Grune and Stratton)

Muller, H.F. (1978). The electroencephalogram in senile dementia. In Nandy, K. (ed) *Senile Dementia: A Biomedical Approach.* (Amsterdam: Elsevier North-Holland)

Obrist, W.D. (1978a), Electroencephalography in aging and dementia. In Katzman, R., Terry, R.D. and Bick, K.L. (eds). *Alzheimer's disease: Senile Dementia and Related Disorders.* (New York: Raven Press)

6
Cerebral blood flow in dementia

I send it through the rivers of your blood
Even to the court, the heart, to th' seat o' the brain,
And, through the cranks and offices of man,
The strongest nerves and small inferior veins
From me receive that natural competency whereby they live.
William Shakespeare (1564–1616),
Coriolanus, I.i, 141-146

The role of impaired blood supply in the pathogenesis of the commoner dementias was one of the first aetiological possibilities to interest investigators into the condition. Naturally, with the availability of techniques for the measurement of cerebral blood flow (CBF), the possibility of relating blood flow to the clinical syndrome of dementia and its laboratory correlates has been pursued by various investigators and has promised much at various times.

The results, however, have not been unequivocal and, given the nature of technical difficulties, this is hardly surprising. Until recently, moreover, distinction between the different groups of dementia in which CBF has been studied has been made solely on clinical grounds, and this again has almost certainly been a fruitful source of error in much earlier work. Again, until relatively recently, age and sex corrections, vital one would have thought to any interpretation of a measure of function have not been made. Furthermore, the symptomatology of dementia, e.g. speech disorder, can itself cause changes in blood flow and the separation of this from the aberrations due to underlying pathology is hardly ever made. Recent studies have shown that intellectual activity itself can elevate blood flow. As a cardinal feature of any dementia is the ideational poverty, the effect of this on the flow has to be considered before blood flow can be related to the dementing process itself.

Most studies are carried out with methods which measure the average rates of blood flow and O_2 consumption in the brain as a whole, or in relatively large regions of it. These measures are thus likely to mask the dysfunction arising from minute, discrete areas in the brain, which may well characterize some dementing process.

For these reasons a high degree of scepticism is required at present in evaluating the role of CBF in dementia.

SOME AVAILABLE PROCEDURES

Kety and Schmidt (1945) developed the nitrous oxide method for the quantitative determination of CBF in man. This method provided for the first time the means to measure the blood flow and metabolic rate of the human brain in the normal conscious state and in pathological conditions.

Lassen and Ingvar (1972) based their multi-regional measurements of CBF on the *intra-arterial* xenon-133 technique. A bolus of saline containing the isotope is injected into the internal carotid artery in conjunction with cerebral angiography. A battery of detectors placed at the side of the head records the arrival and subsequent clearance of the isotope. The clearance curve is a function of the blood flow in the region seen by each detector. Multi-detector devices have been designed to yield 'functional landscapes' of the injected hemisphere. The flow values represent the levels of function in different regions of the cerebral cortex. With the aid of computers, 'mean landscapes' can be calculated and these depict the average distribution of function in normal subjects as well as in patients in different diagnostic groups (Ingvar, 1980).

Obrist (1978b) describes the non-invasive xenon-133 *inhalation* method which now provides an opportunity for systematic investigation of ageing and dementia not possible before their advent. The technique is based on the same principle as the original Kety–Schmidt method, i.e. measurement of the brain's uptake and clearance of an inert, diffusible gas. Although similar to the regional cerebral blood flow (rCBF) method of Lassen and Ingvar in its use of xenon-133 as a tracer, it differs from the latter technique in the route of isotope administration. Rather than introducing xenon-133 directly into the internal carotid artery, the isotope is administered either by inhalation or intravenous injection. This has the obvious advantage of avoiding the risk of carotid artery puncture, thus permitting serial determination during the course of a patient's illness plus the collection of adequate normal control data. Because the isotope is delivered by the blood to both hemispheres, simultaneous bilateral as well as regional measurements can be made.

The non-invasive rCBF method, which was first introduced by Veall and Mallett (1966) and further developed by Obrist *et al.* (1975), consists of brief inhalation (or intravenous injection) of xenon-133 with extracranial monitoring of the subsequent clearance, usually for a period of 10–15 minutes. By using multiple small detectors (as many as 8 or 16 over each hemisphere) it is possible to observe both regional and hemisphere differences in blood flow. The clearance curves are subjected to a two-compartmental analysis, using isotope concentration in the end-expired air to estimate and correct for arterial recirculation. Two clearance rates are obtained from which blood flows are computed for a faster-clearing compartment, considered to be grey matter, and a slower-clearing compartment, representing white matter and extracerebral tissue (scalp and calvarium). Although grey and white matter can be clearly differentiated in the normal subject, shifts in the relative clearance rate of these tissues in pathological conditions may lead to a lack of correspondence between blood flow measurements and anatomically defined compartments. This difficulty can be at least partially circumvented by computation of a mean blood flow for all tissues observed by the detector.

A disadvantage of the non-invasive xenon-133 method is the presence of isotope contamination from extracerebral sources that tends to lower the computed blood flow values. Furthermore, the use of end-expired air as an estimate of arterial isotope concentration may distort the results in patients with lung disease. When properly taken into account, however, these limitations appear to be outweighed by the many advantages of the technique (Obrist, 1978b; see also Risberg, 1980; see below).

The parameters commonly used in CBF measurement are as follows (Gustafson, 1979; Yamaguchi et al., 1980):

Flow in grey matter or fast flow   – F_1, F_f, F_g.
Flow in white matter or slow flow – F_2, F_s, F_w.
Initial flow   – F_{init}.
Weight of grey matter   – W_1.

Risberg (1980) has considered some of the limitations of the xenon-133 inhalation technique. He expresses caution as to the sensitivity of this technique in detecting cortical flow changes during sensory activation procedures (see below); also, there is a 'cross-talk' effect, i.e. a detector partially recording radiation originating in the contralateral hemisphere causing an underestimate of true hemispheric flow asymmetries if detectors are placed laterally, the extracranial contamination of the xenon-133 inhalation curves, and the limited and inefficient extent of concentrating the tracer in the brain.

It is necessary to mention briefly the recent introduction of a technique using steady-state oxygen-15 and positron emission tomography for the non-invasive measurement of rCBF and cerebral mean regional O_2 utilization (rCMRO$_2$) (Frackowiak et al., 1980).

Frackowiak et al. (1981) found a decline in CBF and rCMRO$_2$ correlating with increasing severity of dementia in both degenerative and vascular dements. Focal abnormalities in O_2 utilization were observed for both vascular and degenerative groups. In the vascular group parietal defects were the most pronounced. In the degenerative group parietal and temporal defects were seen in the less severe group, but a profound depression in the frontal regions with relative sparing of occipital areas characterized the severe degenerative dements.

The O_2–extraction ratio measures the degree to which tissues remove oxygen. It has been suggested that the O_2-extraction ratio is unchanged in Alzheimer's disease. When tissues are ischaemic, however, a greater amount of oxygen is removed from the blood, so the absence of an increase of the O_2-extraction ratio indicates ischaemia is not part of the process causing Alzheimer's disease (Frackowiak *et al.*, 1981).

Lenzi *et al.* (1977) had used a combination of xenon-133 and oxygen-15 inhalation to show regions where flow exceeded metabolic need (luxury perfusion) and regions where metabolic need exceeded flow (ischaemia). In multi-infarct dementia they could show a low flow which matched oxygen extraction and seemed to be adequate for local metabolic needs. There were no areas of high metabolism with low flow, hence management might be better served by preventing further infarction than by attempting to improve flow by vasodilator drugs.

NORMAL VARIATION

In the normal, conscious, resting state, the distribution of blood flow/function in both hemispheres is very similar (Ingvar, 1980). The blood flow in frontal and pre-central parts of the hemisphere cortex is significantly higher than in post-central parts in parietal, occipital and temporal regions. The ratio in some regions may be 1 to 2. Ingvar (1980) has interpreted this pattern to show that the conscious state of awareness implies a high activity in afferent parts of the cortex which are responsible for programming our behaviour. The low activity in post-central ('afferent') parts of the cortex implies that in the conscious resting state the afferent sensory input might be inhibited. This seems to agree with crude introspective data: while awake and resting in silence, one is not continuously aware of sensory input; at the same time, the conscious mind is busy 'producing' thoughts, including plans for the future based on previous experience.

An augmentation of the sensory input in the form of cutaneous stimulation, auditory impulses or visual stimulation increases brain activity and, hence, also CBF (Ingvar, 1980). The increase is most marked in the primary projection area of the sensory modality stimulated, but there usually is also an increase in blood flow in the frontal parts of the brain. Possibly the frontal activation is an integrative part of the brain activity involved in perception. For example, stimulation with white noise mainly activates the primary auditory regions, while stimulation with a meaningful noise, music or spoken words, activates the frontal lobes as well (Ingvar, 1980).

Voluntary motor activity activates the respective parts of the Rolandic area according to the somatotopic map. The increase in blood flow to the contralateral cortical hand area during one-sided hand movements is substantial, sometimes being more than 100% (Ingvar, 1979; Oleson, 1971). Indeed, specific pure motor ideation without visible movement is accompanied by cortical activation including a frontal blood flow increase (Ingvar and Risberg, 1967).

Speech and reading activate the speech centres of Broca, Wernicke and Penfield in the lower frontal lobe, the posterior temporal lobe and the supplementary motor area respectively (Ingvar and Schwartz, 1974).

Ingvar and Risberg (1965, 1967) first presented evidence that general and localised flow increases occurred when a subject worked on mental tasks during rCBF study.

Age

As Obrist (1978b) has noted, the fact that elderly demented patients have reduced rCBF relative to healthy young adults does not indicate whether the decline in blood flow is due to age *per se* or pathological processes underlying the dementia. Table 6.1 compares healthy young adults with normal and demented elderly subjects using xenon-133 inhalation (Obrist, 1978b, from data by Obrist, 1975 and Wang and Busse, 1975).

Table 6.1 Fast compartment rCBF (parietal region) (after Obrist, 1978b)

Condition	No. of cases	Age (years)	$F_1(ml(100\ g)^{-1}\ min^{-1})$
Normal young	35	23±3	66.4± 8.7
Normal aged	48	80±7	47.4±10.2
Dementia	20	60±9	40.9± 9.8

It can be seen that whereas the demented patients showed a 38% reduction in F_1, the normal aged subjects had a 28% reduction. Clearly, age itself can account for a significant decline in CBF, although not of the same magnitude as that obtained in dementia. Obrist concludes there is a continuum of blood flow changes, ranging from the healthy young adult to elderly demented patients, with normal aged subjects between.

Yamaguchi *et al.* (1980) also believe there is a diffuse and significant reduction in bihemispheric F_1 values with advancing age. This does not appear to include the brain stem–cerebellar regions and F_2 values. The weight of the faster-clearing compartment or W_1 was also significantly reduced in normal ageing but no greater than in dements of the same age. They believe this suggests Alzheimer's disease is primarily a metabolic disorder of neurones reducing grey matter flow, rather than due to an excessive neuronal loss with ageing with secondary reduction of F_1.

The progressive reduction of W_1 with normal ageing is attributed to diffuse hemispheric cortical loss of neurones occurring in normal aged populations at necropsy and recognizable as ventricular enlargement and cortical atrophy on CT studies during life (Yamaguchi *et al.*, 1980).

MENTAL STATUS AND EEG

Studies among demented patients have shown significant correlations between the magnitude of rCBF reduction and the severity of intellectual impairment. Using the xenon-133 inhalation method Wang and Busse (1975) showed that such a relationship could exist even in normal subjects. Table 6.2 presents their findings on a group of 48 community volunteers of mean age 80. The subjects were divided into two groups according to whether their rCBF (F_1) was above or below the median value of the total sample.

The groups differed significantly in performance on the Wechsler Adult

Intelligence Scale (WAIS) and in dominant EEG frequency (occipital alpha rhythm). Performance as opposed to the verbal scale of WAIS was more impaired in the low rCBF group, a finding consistent with higher deterioration quotients in these subjects and EEG frequency was slower in the low blood flow group.

Table 6.2 Normal aged subjects with high and low rCBF (after Obrist, 1978b, from data by Wang and Busse, 1975)

Measurement	High flow (n=24)	Low flow (n=24)
WAIS scaled scores		
Verbal	60 ±21	52 ±21
Performance	32 ±14[*]	24 ±11[*]
Full	92 ±34	77 ±32
Deterioration quotient	0.19± 0.11[**]	0.30± 0.16[**]
EEG frequency (cps)	9.3 ± 0.6[**]	8.5 ± 0.7[**]

[*] $p < 0.05$; [**] $p < 0.05$

Blood pressure (BP)

Wang and Busse (1975) made further observations on the relationship between BP and rCBF in their normal aged sample, which is depicted in Table 6.3

Table 6.3 Relationship between BP and rCBF (after Wang and Busse, 1975)

	Mean arterial BP	$F_1(ml(100 g)^{-1} min^{-1})$
Group I	94	42.3[*]
Group II	95 to 114	47.5
Group III	115	52.5[*]

[*] Statistically significant

These findings are also in agreement with a correlation of +0.60 between BP and CBF obtained by Hedlund et al. (1964) on patients with cerebrovascular disease and dementia.

This raises the possibility of defective autoregulation in normal and demented elderly subjects. Obrist (1978b) quotes two studies in which BP was deliberately manipulated whilst CBF was being measured. Simard et al. (1971) found intact autoregulation in middle-aged and elderly demented patients, although only one patient with vascular disease was studied. On the other hand, Bentson et al. (1975) observed a loss of autoregulation in long-term diabetics.

ALZHEIMER'S DISEASE AND VASCULAR (MULTI-INFARCT) DEMENTIA

O'Brian and Mallett (1970) first suggested CBF studies might distinguish between these two major forms of dementia. Using the inhalation xenon-133 method, they measured cortical perfusion rates, in a group of demented patients in whom primary neuronal degeneration was distinguished from degeneration secondary to cerebrovascular disease on the basis of clinical features. They found CBF to be normal in the primary neuronal degeneration group and reduced in the cerebrovascular group. However, as Hachinski (1978) has pointed out, their primary neuronal group did not consist of a single pathological type; patients with Huntington's chorea and motor neurone disease, as well as those with Alzheimer's disease, were included.

Ingvar *et al.* (1978) believe that Alzheimer's disease can be fairly well distinguished from other forms of organic dementia with the aid of clinical, psychiatric and psychometric methods, as well as by rCBF studies and the EEG. In their cases the symptomatology, as well as the rCBF reduction, showed a striking correlation with the distribution of cortical degenerative changes. Another feature of their Alzheimer cases seemed to be the low F_2 and W_1 values, probably related to the marked cortical neuronal loss and ensuing cerebral atrophy in their patients. However Hachinski (1978) found both groups in his series showing a decrease in W_1 compared to controls. He believes that though W_1 cannot be equated exactly with anatomical grey matter because the size of the fast-clearing compartment (W_1) varies with the $PaCO_2$, the functioning grey matter is 'undoubtedly the main contributor' to W_1. The reduction in W_1 may therefore be interpreted as indicating a considerable loss of functioning grey matter relative to white in *both* multi-infarct and primary degenerative dementia. Hachinski's findings are set out in Table 6.4 and discussed further below. In Hachinski's series a significant reduction in mean hemisphere flow was confined to the multi-infarct group, in which it was reflected in all variables except F_2.

Table 6.4 Comparison of mean hemisphere CBF (after Hachinski, 1978)

Variable	Multi-infarct group	Alzheimer group	Control
No. of patients	10	14	5
Age (years)	63	63	43
$PaCO_2$ (mmHg)	43	43	41
F_1 (ml $(100g)^{-1}$ min^{-1})	60[*]	84	91
F_2 (ml $(100g)^{-1}$ min^{-1})	19	24	24
F_{init} (ml $(100g)^{-1}$ min^{-1})	41[*]	57	68
W_1%	43[**]	42	49

[*] $p < 0.01$; [**] $p < 0.05$ comparison with controls

Hachinski's explanation for the difference in flow between the two groups is that although the amount of grey matter is reduced in the primary degenerative group, as indicated by reduction of W_1, the flow through the remaining tissue remains normal. Because CBF is measured in terms of perfusion per 100 g of brain per minute, a generalized loss of brain substance should not reduce the flow, providing the metabolic demands of the remaining brain are normal or near normal.

Ingvar (1980) lists the main CBF findings in Alzheimer's disease as follows:

(1) The hemisphere mean blood flow is reduced commensurate with intellectual deficit.

(2) Regional blood flow reductions correlate with psychometric deficits. Thus, memory deficits correlate with a low blood flow in temporal regions; agnosia and 'confusion' show a parieto-occipito-temporal flow decrease. The most marked deficits seem to be found in patients in whom the reduction also involves the frontal lobes.

(3) Specific blood flow patterns seem to distinguish Alzheimer's disease from Pick's disease. In the latter, the flow reduction is more pronounced in frontal and temporal regions while in Alzheimer's the lowest flows are recorded post-centrally in the parieto-occipito-temporal region.

(4) Speech disturbances also correlate with blood flow abnormalities. Anterior flow reduction shows more expressive aphasia defects, while posterior reductions may show symptoms of receptive aphasia. If the flow is reduced generally, language may be completely lost or highly disorganized.

(5) Autopsy findings demonstrate a clear relationship between regions of low flow and regions with marked neurone loss. However, autopsy findings also show that mesial structures, especially the hippo-campus, may be heavily involved in Alzheimer's disease but these structures are not seen by blood flow techniques which mainly record the flow in the lateral aspects of the hemisphere.

In Alzheimer's disease the rCBF reduction, which appears to be diffuse, bihemispheric and symmetrical, also correlates well with the duration and severity of the dementia (Yamaguchi et al., 1980). They also observe that hemispheric blood flow in the cortex in Alzheimer's disease seemed to decrease before cortical atrophy is measurable as judged by W_1 values or on CT brain scan, suggesting a biochemical or metabolic disorder of neurones and/or synaptic function precedes neuronal loss and that the process is independent of vascular disease, since CBF can be restored temporarily to normal levels by 5% CO_2 inhalation.

Yamaguchi et al. (1980) have also observed that the controversy in the literature between Alzheimer's disease and multi-infarct dementia in terms of rCBF may be attributed to lack of suitable numbers of both kinds of dementia and age-matched normal volunteer controls, a consequence of the invasive methods employed. Another cause has been the failure to separate Alzheimer's disease from multi-infarct dementia on clinical, pathological and CT grounds.

Hachinski et al. (1975) noted rCBF was normal in primary degenerative dementia of the Alzheimer type but was low in multi-infarct dementia. Yamaguchi et al. (1980) found they agreed more with Simard et al. (1971), who reported rCBF in Alzheimer's disease is lower than in those with vascular disease. Yamaguchi et al. (1980) agree that this reduction involves both hemispheres equally.

In the Yamaguchi *et al.* (1980) series of moderately severe cases of multi-infarct dementia, the reduction of rCBF was patchy, bilateral and did not correlate with the severity or duration of dementia. Tomlinson and Henderson (1976) had reported from clinical and neuropathological observation that in multi-infarct dementia, even if the total quantity of destroyed tissue was not gross, dementia might appear when particularly important parts of the brain are destroyed. Yamaguchi *et al.* (1980) conclude from this that the dementia associated with vascular disease requires bilateral patchy lesions located in strategic distributions affecting higher cortical function, most commonly in the middle cerebral artery distribution (temporal, parietal and posterior frontal regions), and that overall reduction of hemispheric blood flow correlates poorly with the severity of dementia.

In multi-infarct dementia there were no regions showing consistent regional F_1 reductions, as patchy regional reductions varied from case to case, often with a bordering zone of relative hyperaemia (Yamaguchi *et al.*, 1980). In their patients with combined Alzheimer's disease and multi-infarct dementia, significant regional reductions were found in the left precentral, left posterior temporal, right parietal, right occipital and right inferior temporal regions. In patients with Alzheimer's disease alone, a significant reduction in F_1 values was found in the left frontal region, along with diffuse bilateral hemispheric reduction, compared with age-matched control subjects.

Yamaguchi *et al.* (1980) also found no significant difference between left and right mean hemispheric F_1 values in their three groups of Alzheimer, multi-infarct and mixed patients, and this seemed to confirm that dementia is a bilateral hemispheric disorder. Neither were the speech areas of the left or speech-dominant hemisphere more severely involved than the right in the three groups of demented patients.

Even if it is accepted that there is reduced flow in multi-infarct dementia, the interpretation of this is difficult. Is this reduced flow the cause, or consequence, of the process underlying the dementia? Ingvar (1979) believes the normal or near-normal reactivity of cerebral vessels to CO_2 changes indicates that it is not generalized loss of reactivity to CO_2 in these cases that is responsible for the low flow. Pathological studies show multiple, small infarcts to be the cause of the associated atrophy. Infarcted tissue is rarely completely unperfused; the level of perfusion, however, is much below that of normal tissue. It seems possible that the low flow per 100 g of brain per minute is because an appreciable portion of each 100 g is infarcted tissue rather than metabolically active cells. The vessels seem capable of supplying more blood but there is no demand. The cause of multiple infarcts in the first instance does not seem to be reduced flow because of loss of vascular reactivity but multiple occlusions of vessels. The possibility that the ischaemic brain contains not only infarcted and normal tissue but also a varying amount of under-perfused tissue must also be kept in mind. Several areas of the brain may also have lost their autoregulation and be sensitive to changes in systemic blood pressure and cardiac function. Areas of viable but functionless cerebral tissue may exist in the acute phase of cerebral infarction but there is no evidence that the under-perfused cerebral tissue can remain dormant for months and years. Most precariously supplied cerebral tissue either dies or recovers, depending on a complex interplay of collateral blood flow, local tissue demand, cerebral oedema and a number of still unknown facts.

OTHER CAUSES OF DEMENTIA

As has been mentioned, low rCBF in Pick's disease is typically found symmetrically distributed in the fronto-temporal areas (Gustafson, 1979). Ingvar *et al.* (1978) note these patients show none of a frontal syndrome but their EEGs are well preserved. The F_2 and W_1 values in cases of Pick's disease are within normal limits, a feature they believe further distinguishes this group from Alzheimer's disease.

Ingvar (1980) also notes that in post-traumatic dementia caused by severe head injuries following, e.g., traffic accidents, very low blood flows may be recorded in certain cortical regions in such cases, and speculates that dead neurones may have been replaced by gliotic scars.

In the apallic state which may develop following severe brain anoxia resulting from cardiac arrest (Ingvar *et al.*, 1978) patients lose their cerebral cortex almost entirely, and may survive with a functioning brain stem and spinal cord for months or years. They show no higher function, the blood flows recorded over the brain are extremely low (10–20% of the normal) and activation patterns (see below) are lost.

Although all patients with Down's syndrome older than age 40 are said to show neuropathological changes similar to those found in Alzheimer's disease (Jarvis, 1948), in the Ingvar *et al.* (1978) series of 12, though half the patients were over 40 years old, only normal CBF and regional variations were seen. Another interesting finding was that results from a psychometric investigation showed no correlation with rCBF, a finding very different from that found in Alzheimer's disease. The low IQ in Down's syndrome is, of course, primarily due to severe subnormality and this conceptual distinction from dementia is considered in Chapter 2.

In normal pressure hydrocephalus, patients have a low CBF mean hemisphere level as well as regional reductions in frontal, and especially in post-central, parieto-occipito-temporal regions (Ingvar *et al.*, 1975). In these cases psychometry may assist in facilitating the differential diagnosis in early cases (Gustafson and Hagberg, 1978).

Yamaguchi *et al.* (1980) believe the diffuse cortical and subcortical lesions of white matter in long-standing multiple sclerosis may produce dementia resulting from disconnection syndromes associated with inter-ruption of inter-hemispheric and intra-hemispheric connections. This results in reduced F_2 in demented patients with multiple sclerosis who have an inability to increase this flow during attempts at behavioural activation.

Gustafson (1979) gained the impression from a preliminary analysis of 200 cases of suspected organic brain disorders that rCBF data are useful in distinguishing 'pseudo-dementia' due to affective disorders. In depressive states, the general as well as regional rCBF values are generally found to be within the normal range (Silfverskiold *et al.*, 1979).

In chronic alcoholism the reduction in blood flow is diffuse and lacks focal features. If the alcohol abuse is discontinued the flow reduction may be reversed to some extent. In addition, it has been found that, in contrast to Alzheimer disease patients, mental activation can cause a flow increase of a fairly normal type in alcoholics (Ingvar *et al.*, 1975; Hagberg, 1978).

Severity and duration

It is interesting to ask if the severity and duration of dementia are reflected in CBF values. Gustafson (1979) has said that in the early stages of Alzheimer's disease, though the general level of blood flow can be normal, there may be diminished post-central distribution. In the Yamaguchi *et al.* (1980) series the severity of dementia correlated directly with mean reduction of bihemispheric F_1 values. In Alzheimer's disease, F_1 values in patients with mild dementia were significantly higher than those with moderate to severe dementia. In all groups with mild dementia, there was no significant difference for bihemispheric F_1 values compared with age-matched healthy control subjects although there was a reduction when compared with young healthy normal subjects.

As for duration, the same authors (Yamaguchi *et al.*, 1980) have shown that in patients with Alzheimer's disease mean bihemispheric F_1 values showed a progressive decrease correlating directly with the duration of dementia. No such correlation was found in multi-infarct dementia, which is in keeping with episodic natural history of multi-infarct dementia without a steadily progressive course.

CT SCAN

The relationship between CBF and EEG has already been touched upon. As for CT, Yamaguchi *et al.* (1980) found that mean hemispheric F_1 values in patients with Alzheimer's disease or with mixed Alzheimer–multi-infarct dementia were more reduced in cases with marked cerebral atrophy determined by CT, compared with those with mild or no atrophy.

Gustafson (1979) has noted a generally close relationship between degenerative cortical changes, the focal or general rCBF abnormalities and psychiatric symptoms. However, in patients with severe degenerative brain stem lesions, a diffuse rCBF reduction could be found without corresponding severe loss of cortical neurones.

Age-relations

Yamaguchi *et al.* (1980) were particularly exercised by age-related controls in their analysis. They found that in none of their demented patients was the slower-clearing, primarily white matter flow (F_2) significantly reduced compared with normal young control subjects. In their series there was no significant reduction of mean F_1 values in patients with multi-infarct dementia compared with age-matched control subjects. Age-related controls would seem crucial in what is after all a physiological variable as well, but up to now largely lip service and sops in the form of CBF in young normal

105

volunteers (when the majority of demented patients are elderly) have been available. No future assessment of any value of CBF in dementia seems possible if this basic variable is not taken into account in the presentation of results.

CO_2 responsiveness

Yamaguchi *et al.* (1980) also showed that in patients with mixed Alzheimer's and multi-infarct dementia, values for CO_2 responsiveness were reduced, as were those for multi-infarct dementia alone. Their two cases of vascular dementia without cerebral atherosclerosis, however, showed normal CO_2 responsiveness. They believe the relatively excessive cerebral vasomotor responsiveness to CO_2 in patients with Alzheimer's disease is attributed to the comparatively low F_1 values in the steady state presumably due to reduced glucose oxidative metabolism of cortical neurones and reduced cortical CO_2 production. They conclude that vasodilator response to hypercapnia appears to be a useful diagnostic test for separating atherosclerotic multi-infarct dementia from Alzheimer's disease.

Behavioural activation

Ingvar *et al.* (1975) found activation procedures carried out in Alzheimer patients showing a subnormal flow at rest changed their rCBF pattern only slightly. They concluded that dementia of the Alzheimer type is accompanied by low activity in the association cortex and a reduced ability to activate these regions during mental effort (Ingvar *et al.*, 1975).

In the Yamaguchi *et al.* (1980) series behavioural activation tested in all types of severe dementia failed to produce significant increase in any rCBF region. In contrast, standard behavioural activation in age-matched normal volunteers resulted in significant mean hemispheric and brainstem–cerebellar F_1 increase of 12.5%.

Some demented individuals show regional reductions of flow instead of the expected increase. These reductions have been attributed to a shunting of rCBF or 'steal' to an association cortex during mental activity. In the Yamaguchi *et al.* (1980) series, in Alzheimer's disease patients, no significant increase in rCBF was seen to accompany the rCBF reductions during behavioural activation, so a steal phenomenon cannot be invoked. In their series the brainstem–cerebellar regions also failed to show any F_1 increase during standard tests of behavioural activation. The authors take this to indicate that the reticular activating system (RAS) fails to become activated in demented subjects during behavioural activation as probably occurs in healthy age-matched normal control subjects. Thus, they felt, part of the failure of hemispheric F_1 increases during standard behavioural activation testing may be due to a loss or diminution of a general arousal response in demented aged people. In addition, disconnection syndromes, as exemplified by demented multiple sclerosis patients, appear to contribute to this failure of the rCBF response during behavioural activation (Yamaguchi *et al.*, 1980).

106

Psychometry

The degree and type of cognitive reduction defined psychometrically showed a specific relationship to general as well as to focal rCBF changes (Hagberg and Ingvar, 1976).

General symptomatology

The range of symptomatology to be found in the dementias has been discussed in Chapters 2 and 3. It is interesting to speculate if the symptoms *per se* can influence rCBF without reference to the underlying pathology. Gustafson (1979) shows a strong relation between pronounced mental deterioration and rCBF reduction in the post-central temporo-parieto-occipital area. He also correlates paranoid symptoms with low posterior temporal and higher frontal flow values, and different types of speech disturbance have been shown to relate to the distribution of rCBF abnormalities in the dominant hemisphere (Gustafson *et al.*, 1978).

When receptive speech disturbances dominated in cases of pre-senile dementia, marked flow reductions were found in post-central and especially in temporo-parietal regions. When expressive speech disturbances dominated, marked frontal and anterior temporal flow reductions were found. In general, the receptive type of speech abnormality was found in Alzheimer's disease and the expressive in the Pick group. However, in none of the cases studied for speech disability could classical focal types of aphasia be demonstrated of the type found in cerebrovascular lesions (Gustafson *et al.*, 1978).

Studying memory function in 16 patients with dementia, Hagberg (1978) demonstrated that verbal memory decreased when the blood flow in temporal and parietal areas was reduced. Spatial recognition correlated with the temporal and lower frontal regions. Other memory tests correlated with temporal region flows only.

SUMMARY

(1) All CBF results must be interpreted with caution and scepticism. Apart from technical difficulties, diagnostic methods have varied and attention has not always been paid to controlling age, sex and severity of dementia. Symptoms of dementia themselves correlate with rCBF, and this rather than underlying pathology may well cause CBF changes.

(2) The two methods in popular use at present are the intra-arterial and inhalation xenon-133 techniques, the latter having the considerable advantage of not being invasive.

(3) In the normal resting state the blood flow in frontal and pre-central parts of the hemisphere cortex is significantly higher than in post-central parts, in parietal, occipital and temporal regions.

(4) Sensory stimulation increases CBF in both the sensory cortex and frontal parts of the brain, in the normal brain.

107

(5) In the normal state, voluntary motor activity, pure motor ideation, speech and reading and mental activity also lead to increased CBF.

(6) There seems to be a continuum of blood flow changes with age, ranging from the healthy young adult to elderly demented patients, with normal aged subjects in between. The weight of the compartment of the brain that gives rise to the fast component of CBF (W_1) is reduced with age. This is generally taken to correspond to grey or neuronal matter.

(7) There also seems to be a relationship between CBF and IQ in normal subjects. This relationship extends to a correlation with the alpha rhythms of the EEG.

(8) Another correlation in normals is between mean arterial BP and CBF, the highest flows being found where mean arterial BP >115 mmHg.

(9) A summary of findings in various types of dementia is given in Table 6.5.

Table 6.5 Summary of CBF findings in dementia

Alzheimer's disease
1. There is a diffuse, bihemispheric and symmetrical reduction in CBF.
2. Lowest flows are recorded post-centrally in the parieto-occipito-temporal region.
3. Reduced rCBF is commensurate with lowered IQ.
4. Reduced rCBF correlates with features such as memory deficit, agnosia and speech disturbances.
5. There is correlation with severity and duration.
6. Reduced fast flow (F_1) is related to marked atrophy on CT.
7. CO_2 responsiveness is relatively preserved.
8. There is little increase in rCBF with behavioural activation.

Pick's disease
1. Flow reduction is most pronounced in frontal temporal regions.
2. Values for slow flow (F_2) and the fast flow compartment (W_1) are intact.

Multi-infarct dementia
1. Reduction of rCBF seems to be patchy, bilateral and does not correlate with the severity or duration of dementia.
2. There is no consistent reduction of regional fast flow (F_1) values.
3. CO_2 responsiveness reduced.

Head injury
Very low blood flow may be recorded in the region of injury.

Normal pressure hydrocephalus
Low CBF hemispheric levels, as well as regional reductions in frontal and especially in post-central parieto-occipito-temporal regions, are found.

'Pseudo-dementia'
In depressive states leading to this, general as well as rCBF values are generally found to be normal.

Further reading

(A full list of references is given at the back of the book.)

Hachinski, V.C. (1978). Cerebral blood flow: differentiation of Alzheimer's disease from multi-infarct dementia. In Katzman, R., Terry, R.D. and Bick, K.L. (eds). *Alzheimer's Disease: Senile Dementia and Related Disorders*. (New York: Raven Press)

Ingvar, D.H. (1980). Regional cerebral blood flow and psychopathology. In Cole, J.O. and Barrett, J.E. (eds) *Psychopathology in the Aged*. (New York: Raven Press)

Obrist, W.D. (1978b). Non-invasive studies of cerebral blood flow in aging and dementia. In Katzman, R., Terry, R.D. and Bick, K.L. (eds). *Alzheimer's Disease: Senile Dementia and Related Disorders*. (New York: Raven Press)

Yamaguchi, F., Meyer, J.S., Yamamoto, M., Sakai, F. and Shaw, T. (1980). Non-invasive regional cerebral blood flow measurements in dementia. *Arch. Neurol.*, 37, 410-418

7
Computerized tomography in dementia

Cast a cold eye
On life, on death
W.B. Yeats (1865–1939)

The revolution wrought in the methods of neurological investigation by computerized tomography (CT) is well acknowledged. The CT scanner, based on the linkage of the X-ray beam, the gamma camera and the computer has been described as the most important addition to the diagnostic armamentarium since Roentgen's X-ray (Cloe, 1976).

Gawler (1981) has given a simple and clear account of the basic technique involved in the CT scanning of the brain. A standard computerized brain scan provides a three-dimensional display of the intracranial anatomy built up from a vertical series of transverse axial tomograms. Each tomogram represents a horizontal slice through the patient's head, reconstructed in terms of the X-ray density of the structures it contains. The technique is sufficiently sensitive to distinguish brain tissue from CSF so that the ventricular system and many of the subarachnoid cisterns are visible. The lateral, third and fourth ventricles are regularly seen but the aqueduct is normally too fine to resolve (see Fig. 7.1).

CT detects the slight difference in X-ray absorption between grey and white matter, and thus allows certain cerebral structures to be identified in their own right.

The primary output of the scanner is in the form of a numerical matrix which can be reconstructed as a pictorial representation, i.e. the photographic scan that comes to the clinician's hand. The traditional method of interpretation is from this picture, and apart from lesions in the substance of the brain, the two common indices studied are cerebral atrophy and ventricular dilation.

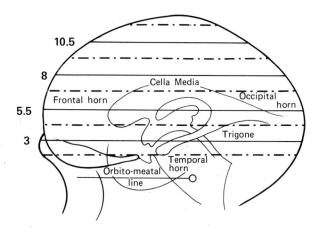

Figure 7.1 The CT head scan. Scan pairs are obtained at 3, 5.5, 8 and 10.5 cm above the orbito-meatal line, thus providing a vertical series of eight tomogram (after Gawler, 1981)

Cerebral atrophy

Gawler (1981) describes cerebral atrophy as being due to a diffuse loss of brain tissue. It is recognized by demonstrating enlargement of cortical sulci or dilation of the ventricular systems. These findings usually coexist but some patients have sulcal dilation in isolation (cortical atrophy) while others show a non-obstructed dilated ventricular system with normal sulci (central atrophy). As Gawler points out further, it is important to realize that cerebral atrophy is not a diagnosis, merely the visible end-point of a spectrum of brain diseases and insults.

The unfortunate confusion between cerebral atrophy and dementia, which tends to prevail in some quarters even today, seems to have arisen in curious circumstances. Until CT became available in the mid-1970s the only method available for the demonstration of atrophic brain change was pneumencephalography (PEG) or air encephalography (AEG). Because the procedure caused discomfort and was attended by risks, it tended to be used only in a minority of neurological patients who presented with rather specific problems, and in whom the exclusion of lesions was as important as the diagnosis. One category so investigated were those presenting with intellectual deterioration, and dementia soon became associated with cerebral atrophy (Gawler, 1981).

As soon as CT was introduced it became clear that the method demonstrated cerebral atrophy. Comparative studies (e.g. Gawler *et al.*, 1976) showed that CT and PEG were equally reliable in this context. Moreover, the CT scan could demonstrate the ventricular system, cortical sulci and subarachnoid space in an undisturbed condition, so avoiding the distortions in ventricular size and sulcal appearances which were known to complicate PEG. For this reason the CT scan was particularly helpful in demonstrating both generalized atrophy and focal atrophy.

The CT scan appearances of cerebral atrophy include enlargement of the cortical sulci, and Gawler goes on to advise it is essential to obtain a vertex slice as the most prominent sulci may be apparent only at this level. Widening of the interhemispheric fissure, and enlargement of the insular cisterns on each side, are further indications of cerebral atrophy on computerized scans (Gawler, 1981).

Jacoby *et al.* (1980) describe a simple method for rating cortical atrophy. A cortical atrophy score is given by an experienced neuro-radiologist after he has rated the ventricular system as small, normal or enlarged. The cortical atrophy score is given on a four-point scale (none, mild, moderate, severe) for five cortical regions (frontal, parietal, temporal, insulae, occipital). The maximum possible score is 20 (4 × 5). On this basis the mean score for their sample of 50 normal subjects of mean age 73 years was 2.0±1.79 with a range from 0 to 7.

Because there is no risk with CT it has allowed study of the cerebral anatomy in patients with a wide range of neurological disease including those such as migraine, where cerebral pathology is not anticipated. These studies have shown cerebral atrophy to be fairly common, particularly in older patients, and it is now clear that the finding does not necessarily indicate a dementing illness (Gawler, 1981). Thus cerebral atrophy is a fairly common finding among those who present with epilepsy of late onset but psychometric evaluation in such patients is often normal. Claveria *et al.* (1977) have also drawn attention to the poor correlation between mental function and CT appearances of cerebral atrophy. Thus intellectual function may be well preserved in patients who show fairly gross atrophy, while some patients with severe dementia have normal scans. Although it may be possible to show a broad correlation between the degree of ventricular dilatation and the level of intellectual impairment, it is important to underline that for an individual patient the demonstration of mild or moderate atrophy does not necessarily indicate a disease which will lead to progressive intellectual failure.

Soininen *et al.* (1981), studying normals, found cortical atrophy in the left temporal region correlated with the low psychological test score. This may be related to asymmetric findings in the left temporal region in the EEG, which are common in normal elderly people. It has been suggested that this atrophy in the left temporal region in clinical normals may be related to 'benign senescent forgetfulness' (Kral, 1978).

Ventricular dilatation

Measurement of ventricular enlargement, it has been suggested (Donaldson, 1979), may be of value in the clinical staging of the disease and perhaps in early diagnosis. Ventricular size is comparatively easy to measure and various methods and ventricular indices have been advocated (Fig. 7.2).

Evans' Ratio
ratio of maximal width of frontal horns
of the lateral ventricle to the maximum
internal diameter of the skull.

Cella media index
ratio of minimal width of lateral
ventricles in cella media region and
respective width of outer skull table.

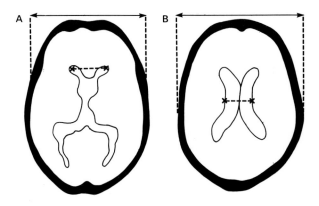

Figure 7.2   Two measurements of ventricular dilatation (modified from Soininen *et al.*, 1982)

Evans' ratio, originally established for the estimation of ventricular enlargement on PEG is one such measure (see Figure 7.2).

Barron *et al.* (1976) studied ventricular size during ageing and found a gradual, progressive increase in ventricular size from first to sixth decade followed by a dramatic increase in the eight and ninth decades. The range of normal ventricular size was relatively wider in the eight and ninth decades than in the first seven. This was more or less confirmed by Gyldensted (1977), who found measurements of the various parts of the ventricular system showing an increase with age and also showing a sex difference.

Two planimetric measures of ventricular size are described by Synek and Reuben (1976) and Jacoby *et al.* (1980).

Jacoby *et al.* (1980) also described CT and brief psychometric findings on 50 psychiatrically and neurologically healthy community residents over 60 years. A reciprocal relationship was found between a global rating of cortical atrophy and a test of memory and orientation among the normal elderly. The significance of this is taken up later in relation to the discussion on dementia.

Numerical interpretation of the data

It has already been said that the conventional study of the CT scan is based on the photographic plate that is reconstructed from the basic numerical data. But attention has increasingly been paid to study of the numbers themselves.

A Hounsfield Unit (HU) is equivalent to a CT number or CT value. It is

114

related to the coefficient of attenuation of brain material within the voxel (see Fig. 7.4) under the condition of scanning at the location.

A very rough guide to the kind of attenuation densities studied has been compiled from several sources and is given in Fig. 7.3.

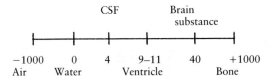

Figure 7.3   Attenuation densities in Hounsfield Units or CT numbers (after several authors)

The mean HU (or CT) value of a unit volume of brain tissue (voxel) is related to tissue density, which depends on chemical composition and reflects the X-ray attenuation coefficient of tissue components. In CT scans of the quality produced by routine scanning techniques, normal brain tissue is readily differentiated from localized areas of greater or lesser density due, for example, to defective myelination, the accumulation of abnormal products of metabolism and the abnormal accumulation of blood. However, the capacity of the CT scanner to detect localized areas of altered tissue density may be limited by technical artefacts (Bondareff *et al.*, 1981).

A further methodological problem in the analysis of CT scans is that of deciding upon the ventricular boundary (Jacoby *et al.*, 1980). Because each slice is 10–13 mm thick (depending on the generation of the scanner) and because the ventricular system is complex in shape, many *pixels* (see Fig. 7.4) at the brain–ventricle interface will have an absorption density which is partly due to brain tissue and partly to CSF, the anatomical area represented by such pixels being occupied by both brain and CSF. This phenomenon is termed *partial volume artefact* and is also illustrated in Figure 7.4 (Jacoby *et al.*, 1980).

Thus, if the numerical scan data are used the absorption density is taken and all pixels at or below the number in the centre of the slice are counted as ventricle.

The interpretation of numerical data in CT scans taken in dementia patients is a promising departure, and is considered in somewhat greater detail in the next section.

CT in dementia

Perhaps the most important present-day use of the CT scan in dementia is for the exclusion of causes of dementia other than those leading to primary degenerative disease. Displacement and deformity of the ventricular system is usually clearly evident in these cases and abnormal tissue attenuation, with increased attenuation after the introduction of contrast, will reveal most tumours. Occasional difficulty may arise in the presence of isodense

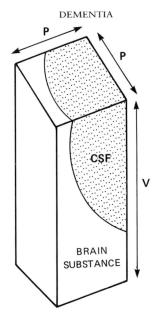

Figure 7.4 Partial volume artefact. Diagrammatic representation of a single pixel/voxel of the CT scan matrix occupied by both brain substance and CSF (after Jacoby *et al.*, 1980)

(A *pixel* is a single picture element cell in the matrix 160 × 160 which is the standard output of most CT scanners. It is the two-dimensional representation of the scanned volume element (voxel).)

$p \times p = $ pixel
$p \times p \times v = $ voxel

subdural haematoma and normal pressure hydrocephalus is not readily diagnosed by CT scan (Donaldson, 1979). Jacobs *et al.* (1976) and Kinkel and Jacobs (1976) consider the CT to be excellent in excluding vascular and expanding lesions.

The value of the CT was considered by Du Boulay *et al.* (1975) in an evaluation of 107 patients considered to be demented on clinical evaluation. Table 7.1 gives a summary of their findings.

Given the interest in cerebral atrophy and ventricular dilatation from the days of PEG, it was only natural that these indices be sought on CT and an attempt made to relate them to clinical findings. There has been much conflicting data and a good deal of confusion though an attempt has been made in Table 7.2 to provide a summary of findings and conclusions. One of the major difficulties has been the lack of suitable normative data. 'Normal' controls have been taken on occasion (Roberts and Caird, 1976) to mean patients with 'minor degrees of memory impairment'. Others have used patients with headache (Gyldensted, 1977) and normal elderly persons able to live independently in the community (Gonzalez *et al.*, 1978).

Table 7.1   CT evaluation in patients with dementia (after du Boulay *et al.*, 1975)

	Abnormality on CT scan	Normal CT scan
Dementia unrelated to specific disease (senile dementia)	35	3
Dementia associated with specific disease (chiefly cerebrovascular disease, alcoholism, Parkinson's disease, malignant disease, previous head injury, chronic epilepsy, Huntington's chorea, hypothyroidism)	48	3
Hydrocephalus	5	
Tumour	4	
Infarct	4	
Psychiatric disease	0	5
Total	96	11

It almost goes without saying that pathology, including the serious kind that produces dementia, cannot be excluded from any of these groups, and they cannot be considered suitable controls.

It has come to be noted that when groups of demented patients are studied by CT they are seen to exhibit significantly more atrophy than controls, but dementia occurs without atrophy and atrophy without dementia. In one study 16% of controls were found on blind rating to have enlarged ventricles, whereas 25% of dements had normal ventricles (Jacoby and Levy, 1980). When it came to the symptoms of dementia, Soininen *et al.* (1982), in a study of 57 patients with senile dementia, found cortical atrophy did not correlate with psychological test score.

While cortical atrophy shows no significant correlation with intellectual impairment in *demented* patients, a striking finding (e.g. Jacoby *et al.*, 1980; Soininen *et al.*, 1982) has been the discovery that in *normal* controls cortical atrophy related to lower scores on cognitive testing. In the Soininen *et al.* (1982) series there was particular correlation with atrophy in the left temporal region. Jacoby *et al.* (1980) suggest two possibilities in explanation. One is that the type of non-progressive cognitive impairment sometimes found in normal elderly subjects and described by Kral (1962) as 'benign senescent forgetfulness' may have a structural basis. The other is that some of the subjects tested were in fact very early cases of senile dementia.

Another interesting finding (Jacoby and Levy, 1980) is that there is an inverse relationship between cortical atrophy and paranoid delusions, implying the capacity for paranoid ideation, which is at least in part an intellectual phenomenon, is incompatible with severe cortical atrophy.

Fox *et al.* (1975) had noted that senile dementia patients with moderate or severe atrophy had a poorer short-term prognosis than those with uncertain or mild atrophy. In a more specific attempt to relate atrophy to prognosis Jacoby and Levy (1980) believe that subjects with marked parietal atrophy on CT have a significantly shorter life expectancy, which seems to confirm suspicions raised by earlier clinical and neuropathological work.

Fox *et al.* (1975) tried to make further sense of their subgroup with minimal atrophy. Finding two patients with potentially treatable illnesses (hypothyroidism and pernicious anaemia) and questionable atrophy on CT, they wondered if patients with dementia but relatively little atrophy on CT represented a unique group with a better prognosis who require particularly careful evaluation for potentially treatable illness. But this promising impression has not been consistently borne out by subsequent research.

At the same time as cortical atrophy has been shown not to have a consistent relationship to elements in the dementia syndrome, ventricular enlargement has been found to be a somewhat more significant index. While Jacoby and Levy (1980) found only weakly significant relationships or non-significant trends between psychological impairment and measure of ventricular enlargement in a group of demented patients as compared to healthy controls and depressed patients, Soininen *et al.* (1982) found several measures of ventricular dilatation increased with intellectual impairment in their series.

However, Jacoby and Levy (1980) also found that demented patients under 80 had significantly larger ventricles than those of 80 years and over, which led them to ask if early-onset dementia might be a more malignant condition. They also considered the significance of the correlation of their cortical atrophy score with a planimetric measure of ventricular area in controls, but not in cases of dementia, and believe this might offer some support for the view that the atrophic process in senile dementia is fundamentally different from the atrophy associated with normal ageing. This finding also seems to suggest that in senile dementia, cortical atrophy and ventricular dilatation operate to some extent independently of each other.

In an effort to compare cerebral blood flow and CT, Melamed *et al.* (1978) measured regional cerebral blood flow (rCBF) by the xenon-133 inhalation method in 25 patients with dementia who underwent CT. There was no correlation between rCBF and the severity of ventricular dilatation or cortical atrophy. The authors suggest this might indicate that a loss of brain substance is not an important factor in the reduction of rCBF in dementia.

Findings somewhat at odds with those in the foregoing paragraphs were reported by George *et al.* (1981), who demonstrated a correlation between loss of grey–white matter discriminability and cognitive impairment. Their patients with the most severe cognitive impairment demonstrated virtual isodensity of grey and white tissue. Loss of discriminability correlated with nearly all cognitive measures and also with estimates of ventricular dilatation and cortical atrophy. Whereas previous studies had consistently shown stronger correlations between ventricular enlargement and cognitive impairment, in this study grey–white discriminability loss was correlated more consistently at the cortical level with measures of cognitive impairment.

However, they showed increasing dementia being associated with *increasing* attenuation values for both grey and white matter, and also believed cognitive impairment may be more closely related to the left rather than right hemisphere attenuation changes. This differs somewhat from the reports included in the discussion to follow. George *et al.* (1981) conclude the results of their method, whilst showing a close correlation between grey–white changes and ventricular enlargement, suggest that a relationship may exist between parenchymal and ventricular changes.

Ladurner *et al.* (1982) studied 71 patients with ischaemic stroke, divided into those with and without dementia. CT confirmed the importance of bilateral distribution of infarcts in the demented group. Another finding was the higher distribution of infarcts in the region of the thalamus in the demented group. They also confirmed the importance of infarcts in vascular dementia even when they had been neurologically silent.

On the other hand, when Radue *et al.* (1978) had compared cases with vascular dementia with 'parenchymatous' dementia on clinical grounds and CT features, there was an agreement of only 40% between clinical and radiological diagnosis. This was because 10 out of 19 cases of clinically diagnosed 'multi-infarct' dementia showed no radiological evidence of infarction.

Attenuation coefficients in dementia

Naeser *et al.* (1980) studied white matter in the centrum semiovale slice of the CT and found CT numbers (HU) were higher for six non-dementia cases (CT numbers of 41 and above) than for 14 dementia cases (CT numbers of 40 and below). They felt the differential diagnosis between dementia and depression may be better aided by studying the CT numbers rather than the presence of prominent sulci. They also go on to suggest a possible explanation for these findings. They believe the lower CT numbers (closer to CSF, see Fig. 7.3) in the dementia cases may represent an on-going degenerative process within the grey and/or white matter at the centrum semiovale slice level. It is possible the lower CT numbers reflect degeneration within the white matter that may precede the degeneration of all bodies (cortical grey matter) and development of senile plaques and neurofibrillary tangles. Hence, the lower CT number observations in the white matter could precede the development of prominent sulci in the cortex of dementia cases. The development of prominent sulci in non-dementia cases is probably due to other mechanisms.

Bondareff *et al.* (1981) computed mean CT numbers (or Hounsfield Units) in 15 regions of the brain in CT scans of 25 patients with senile dementia and 29 normal volunteers. Mean CT numbers were significantly lower bilaterally in the medial temporal lobe, anterior frontal lobe and head of the caudate nucleus in the group of patients with senile dementia. There was no correlation between mean CT numbers and age. The authors felt their data suggested that the determination of mean CT numbers from selected technically suitable regions of CT scans of the brain may have clinical application in the diagnosis of senile dementia and provide a reliable means of monitoring changes in brain tissue density during the course of senile dementia.

Naguib and Levy (1982), on following up patients suffering from senile dementia, found measures of ventricular size and cortical atrophy were not of predictive value but measurement of radiological density showed this to be significantly lower in the right parietal region of the CT scans of those who subsequently died. Their study seemed also to confirm further that involvement of the parietal lobes is an indication of poor prognosis.

A further discussion of the role of CT in dementia is available in Jacoby (1982).

A brief word needs to be said about the new technique of proton nuclear magnetic resonance (NMR) in its application to the diagnosis of dementia. A preliminary report (Besson *et al.*, 1983) attempted to distinguish between 'parenchymal' and vascular dementia cases, classified on clinical grounds on the basis of the Hachinski ischaemic score. Both demented groups showed significantly greater spin-lattice relaxation times (T_1) in all white matter areas than the controls, but there was no significant difference between them. In terms of proton density (PD) values, however, these were significantly greater in 'parenchymal' dementia than in vascular or among the controls. These changes were observed even when lesions were not seen on visual inspection of the images, and it is suggested that proton NMR measures on white-matter permit the differentiation of 'parenchymal' (the authors claim these findings are applicable to senile dementia of the Alzheimer type) from vascular dementia and from non-dementia in situations where visual lesions are not detected and where other imaging techniques are inconclusive. Further reports are awaited with interest.

SUMMARY (ALSO SEE TABLE 7.2)

(1) A standard CT scan provides a three-dimensional display of the intracranial anatomy built up from a vertical series of transverse axial tomograms (Fig. 7.1). The primary output of the scanner is numerical and this can be pictorially reconstructed.

(2) The two most important traditional indices from the scan picture are measures of cerebral atrophy and ventricular dilatation.

(3) In the past, for historical reasons, cerebral atrophy was equated with dementia. This is now known not to be invariable.

(4) CT scan appearances of cerebral atrophy include enlargement of the cortical sulci, widening of the inter-hemispheric fissure and enlargement of the insular cisterns.

(5) CT scan appearances of cerebral atrophy are fairly common in normals, especially in older patients.

(6) Evans' ratio and the cella media index are two of several methods adopted for measurement of ventricular dilatation.

(7) Age and sex differences are detectable in measuring ventricular dilatation and have to be controlled.

Table 7.2 Summary of findings in some studies of CT

Study	Type of subject	Conclusions
1. Fox *et al.* (1975)	35 senile dementia patients	Patients with little or no atrophy may have a treatable cause and better prognosis.
2. Roberts and Caird (1976)	66 elderly subjects (17 clinically normal)	Broad relationship between increasing ventricular dilatation and increasing intellectual impairment.
3. Jacoby *et al.* (1980)	50 normals	Considerable overlap in incidence of cerebral atrophy. Ventricular size more important in relation to cognitive impairment in dementia patients. Cortical atrophy more important in normals.
4. Jacoby and Levy (1980)	40 senile dements 41 affectives	
5. Soininen *et al.* (1982)	57 senile dementia patients 85 controls	Measures of ventricular dilatation increased with intellectual impairment but no correlation with cortical atrophy.
6. Naeser *et al.* (1980)	6 non-dements 14 dements	CT numbers higher for non-dementia than for dementia cases.
7. Bondareff *et al.* (1981)	25 senile dementia patients 29 normal volunteers	Mean CT number lower bilaterally in three regions of brain in dements.
8. Naguib and Levy (1982)	40 senile dementia patients	Lower CT numbers in right parietal region predictive of poor prognosis.

(8) A reciprocal relationship is found between cortical atrophy and cognitive measures in the normal elderly. This may provide a basis for 'benign senescent forgetfulness'.

(9) A Hounsfield Unit (HU) is equivalent to a CT number or CT value. It is related to the coefficient of attenuation of brain material within the voxel under the condition of scanning at the location (see Fig. 7.4).

(10) CT scanning in dementia can probably be used for exclusion of causes of dementia and is especially useful in excluding vascular and expanding lesions.

(11) In cases of dementia cortical atrophy does not consistently correlate with psychological test score. However, it has been suggested that those dements who show little or no atrophy may have a treatable cause of dementia and a better prognosis.

(12) It has also been suggested that those who have marked parietal atrophy may have a significantly shorter life expectancy.

(13) Several measures of ventricular enlargement seem to increase with intellectual impairment in demented patients.

(14) Thus cortical atrophy and ventricular dilatation seem to operate independently of one another.

(15) There seems no correlation between regional cerebral blood flow (rCBF) and the severity of ventricular dilatation or cortical atrophy.

(16)However, there seems to be a correlation between loss of discrimination between grey and white matter and cognitive impairment. This correlates in turn with ventricular dilatation and cortical atrophy, and may provide the link between parenchymal and ventricular changes.

(17)CT numbers in certain regions of the brain seem lower in dementia. When reduced in the right parietal region they seemed predictive of poor prognosis.

Further reading

(A full list of references is given at the end of the book)

Bondareff, W., Baldy, R. and Levy, R. (1981). Quantitative computed tomography in dementia. *Arch. Gen. Psychiatry*, **38**, 1365-1368

Gawler, J. (1981). Computed axial tomography of the brain. In Dawson, A.M., Compston, N. and Besser, G.M. (eds). *Recent Advances in Medicine*. Vol 18. (London: Churchill Livingstone)

Jacoby, R.J., Levy, R. and Dawson, J.M. (1980). Computed tomography in the elderly: 1. The normal population. *Br. J. Psychiatry*, **136**, 249-255

Jacoby, R.J., and Levy, R. (1980). Computed tomography in the elderly: 2. Senile dementia: diagnosis and functional impairment. *Br. J. Psychiatry*, **136**, 256-269

Soininen, H., Puranen, M. and Reikkinen, P.J. (1982). Computed tomography findings in senile dementia and normal ageing. *J. Neurol. Neurosurg. Psychiatry*, **45**, 50-54

8
The pathology of dementia

Of its own beauty is the mind diseased.
Lord Byron (1788-1824)

A study of the diverse aspects of the pathological process begins logically with the changes that are undergone by the ageing normal brain. The discussion in this section is based on accounts provided by Armbrustmacher (1979), Tomlinson (1979), Bowen and Davison (1981), and Shaw and Meyer (1982).

The human brain increases four-fold in weight during the first 3 years of life, then steadily to about the age of 18. The first significant signs of decreasing weight are seen about 45 years and the decline continues into the eighties. It is believed that neuronal degeneration and replacement gliosis result in an average reduction in brain weight of 11% over five decades.

Apart from the decrease in brain weight and volume, the most obvious naked-eye change with advancing age is the increasing prominence of gyral atrophy. The greatest loss of weight occurs after the age of 60 in normals but the contribution of various degenerative processes to the picture has to be allowed for to an increasing extent after that age. It has also to be kept in mind that there has been a secular change in human size, analogous to that for cognitive processes, over several generations. Mean human heights have increased over the past 50 years as almost certainly has, as Tomlinson (1979) puts it, mean brain weight. Some loss of brain weight in elderly subjects may therefore simply reflect initially smaller brain weight.

In over 50% of normal old brains variable gyral narrowing with sulcal widening is visible, particularly in the parasagittal frontal and parietal, and lateral frontal and lateral temporal cortex; the occipital cortex and all inferior gyri are much less obviously affected.

Hemisphere volume progressively diminishes from the age of 20 years with a greater fall in men than in women. The loss of brain weight is also greater in males than in females. Further, between 20 and 50 years, grey matter volume falls more than white, but after that more white matter is lost than grey, which workers tend to equate with neuronal loss.

Evidence now exists that cortical neurones, cerebellar Purkinje cells and spinal cord motor neurones are all diminished in normal old age but that various brain stem nuclei have their nerve cells virtually intact throughout life.

As is well know, cells of the central nervous system are at their maximum number at birth. There is then a progressive age-related decrease in cell population which begins about the age of 20–25, the end of the period of growth and maturation.

Some areas of the cortex are affected to a greater degree than others. Neuronal loss is particularly significant in the superior frontal gyrus, the superior temporal gyrus, the full extent of the precentral gyrus and the visual cortex. In frontal and temporal areas this neuronal decrease is approximately 40% by the ninth decade, which it is thought, might account for the benign forgetfulness, slower motor performance and other physiological changes among the normal elderly.

Although neuronal loss occurs in all cortical layers, they are most marked in layers 2 and 4. These two layers of the cortex are the last to appear during development, indicating a possibility that a link might exist between the sequence of appearance of structures in the central nervous system and their ability to withstand the rigours of the normal ageing process.

As we have seen, the brain stem structures are not involved in the process of age-related neuronal loss, with the exception of the *locus coeruleus*. The rate of neuronal loss in the nucleus of this structure is said to parallel the rate of cell loss in the cortex. Since this structure is believed to be involved in the regulation of sleep, this finding is of particular interest with respect to the abnormal sleep patterns including insomnia found among the elderly who generally experience a reduction in the duration of sleep, decreased REM (dream) sleep, dreaming and stage 4 (deep) slow wave sleep (see also Chapter 5 on EEG).

At a more basic level, loss of brain substance is reflected by a decrease in myelin, RNA, sodium and potassium while calcium and iron increase; O_2 consumption, too, decreases with age. As was shown in Chapter 6, xenon-133 inhalation cerebral blood flow studies have shown a gradual reduction in hemispheric weight of grey matter with advancing age in normal healthy adults. The lateral ventricles tend to become enlarged, the cortical gyri narrowed and the sulci enlarged. Ventricular measurements based on CT scanning (see Chapter 7) have revealed a gradual increase in ventricular size, with the greatest increase occurring in the eighth and ninth decades.

Microscopy of cerebral blood vessels suggests there are alterations in the cerebral microvasculature in the form of 'corkscrewing', 'spiralling' and 'coiling' of the perforating cortical arteries, arterioles, capillaries and venules. These alterations seem to occur throughout the cerebral cortex and subcortical matter and become more obvious with each passing decade of life. Naked-eye and miscroscopic observations also reveal increased opacification and loss of tubular resiliency of the vessel walls of all sizes with age.

124

Normal ageing and dementia both show atrophy of the brain with neuronal loss, plaque formation and neurofibrillary degeneration. The discussion in succeeding paragraphs considers the other elements, but it may be noted here that the intra-neuronal accumulation of the pigment lipofuscin is also commonly seen in both groups. The significance of lipofuscin accumulation in relation to normal ageing or dementia is uncertain, as the inferior olivary and dentate nuclei are loaded with lipofuscin from infancy and yet remain well-preserved entities in elderly subjects.

We are now in a position to discuss the status of those microscopic changes which were first noted in brains of demented patients. Their relation to the process of ageing has been a matter of some controversy for many years and although the existence of these features – neurofibrillary tangles, senile plaques and granulovacuolar degeneration – has been known for the better part of this century it is only recently that we have been able to assess their significance in an informed way.

Tomlinson *et al.* (1968) and Tomlinson (1972) have considered the position of neurofibrillary tangles. It has been shown that these tangles are to be found in about 50% of apparently normal individuals in their hippocampus in the fifth decade. By the seventh decade almost 60% of subjects seem to be involved, and in the tenth decade virtually all cases show some tangles. In a study of intellectually well-preserved old people who had been followed up till death, Tomlinson *et al.* (1968) could show that neurofibrillary degeneration was the most frequent change, but only found to be numerous in the anteromedial structures of the temporal lobe, and were either absent or present in only very small numbers elsewhere in the neocortex or in deeper-lying hemisphere or brain stem structures. Within the anterior temporal lobe the change seems to be relatively frequent in normal old age and may be present in many neurones in the amygdaloid nucleus, which probably shows the severest changes, in the pyramidal cells of the hippocampus and the glomerular formations of the subiculum, with occasionally some spread into the hippocampal gyri.

Tomlinson's conclusion is that in more than 100 intellectually well-preserved old subjects no case has been seen with more than a very occasional neurofibrillary tangle in the neocortex.

It was once thought that the senile plaque resulted from degeneration of processes of nerve cells already affected by neurofibrillary degeneration. But all the evidence is against this view as plaques occur throughout the neocortex, often in considerable numbers, in normal old people in the total absence of neurofibrillary degeneration.

The other commonly held view, that amyloid had a primary role in initiating the senile plaque, has also come to be rejected. It now appears that plaques are formed by the progressive distension and abnormalities in nerve terminals, and not through the formation of amyloid fibrils or in any other morphological change in the extracellular constituents of the cortex. But there is at least one type of amyloid which results from antibody–antigen reaction and contains immunoglobulins. It has been postulated in this instance that escape of antigen–antibody complexes from blood vessels into

125

the tissues may damage neurites and initiate the degenerative changes noted above. However, the consensus still appears to be that there is insufficient evidence as yet that the amyloid deposited in the centre of plaques is of immunological origin.

When senile plaques are present in very small numbers in the young normal (i.e. under 60 years), they are to be found in the hippocampus, the hippocampal gyrus or the amygdaloid nucleus. The amygdaloid nucleus appears to be the most severely affected structure in the brain in normal subjects and demented patients, by both senile plaques and neurofibrillary tangles.

A small number of normal subjects possess plaques from the age of 30. By the age of 70, plaques in up to moderate numbers may be present throughout the neocortex in some 65% of normal individuals. Very occasionally intellectually intact old subjects are found to have large numbers of widely scattered senile plaques. This is similar in quantity to that found usually in demented patients. Tomlinson has said this phenomenon separates senile plaque formation in the neocortex from neurofibrillary tangle formation, which in his experience never occurs in profusion in the neocortex in intellectually well-preserved subjects.

Nevertheless, with regard to senile plaques in general, there seems to be a correlation between their number and the degree of dementia until this is severe, when the correlation ceases. When intellectual deterioration not amounting to dementia can be detected, these individuals show a smaller number of senile plaques. And when intellectually well-preserved individuals are considered, senile plaques are seen to occur throughout the neocortex in even smaller numbers.

Granulovacuolar degeneration is rare before the senium but after that occurs with increasing frequency in non-demented old people, and in the ninth decade may be present to some degree in 75% of all cases. In normal subjects, in contrast to Alzheimer's disease patients, the change is usually restricted to the pyramidal cells of Sommer's sector and the adjacent subiculum. In the past 20 years it has also been described as being present in other disease states when it is usually found in the hippocampus.

The limitation in brain function that develops with senescence could be due to actual loss of cells or decreased capacity of the cells to perform certain functions, e.g. decrease in production of RNA may limit the capacity for memory storage. Diminished O_2 consumption is probably a reflection of diminished metabolic activity in the cells. Cells, of course, need not be physically lost but there may be a 'dying-back' degenerative process which might result in the loss of many of the neurone's synaptic connections and this would result in the loss of the integrative function of the hemisphere.

The *locus coeruleus*, situated in the caudal pontine central grey matter, contains noradrenergic projections reaching the neocortex. From middle age there is a fall in number of neurones in this region in some subjects. At the age of 70 the cell count in the region is about half those of younger individuals, and by the eighth and ninth decades it may be down to 30–40%. Small declines are seen with catecholamine concentrations with age. Reduction in noradrenaline is found in the hippocampus and 5-HT in the cingulate gyrus. Monoamine oxidase activity, however, increases in the ageing brain through enhanced activity of the enzyme MAO B. There is also a loss in activity of the dopaminergic system. The correlates of reduced transmitter activity involving these systems may be altered sleep habits, depression and dyskinesia.

The hypothalamus, which counts amongst its hormones oxytocin and vasopressin, shows a reduction in transmitter levels with age. There is considerable interest in this finding as vasopressin has now been incriminated in the memory process.

Tyrosine hydroxylase, glutamate decarboxylase and choline acetyl transferase (CAT) activity generally show a significant decrease with ageing. CAT, which catalyses the formation of acetylcholine, undergoes a reduction to the extent that by the tenth decade its activity is only about 10% of the value for that of the neocortex in the young adult. Further evidence is that blockade of central muscarine receptors can convert the pattern of intellectual performance of young adults to that of elderly subjects. An age-related reduction in muscarine receptor building activity seems to occur in the neocortex of normal elderly subjects.

NORMAL AND PATHOLOGICAL CHANGES IN THE AGED BRAIN

From the foregoing it must be clear that there is a distinction that needs to be attempted between the changes in the normal elderly brain and the effects of pathology on it. No feature of histopathology in a demented brain appears to be pathognomonic or even provides a qualitative distinction from the normal. On the contrary, there appears to be a quantitative relationship between normal senile and pathological changes. Roth (1980) has summarized the evidence, much of which comes from the Newcastle study whose methods featured in some of the paragraphs above.

(1) There seems to be a highly significant correlation between indices of dementia derived during life from psychometric assessments continued to near the time of death and measurements of plaques, neurofibrillary change and granulovacuolar degeneration.

(2) Each of the pathological elements associated with senile dementia of Alzheimer type is present to a limited extent in the brains of mentally well-preserved subjects in old age. In other words there is no qualitative difference but all the changes found in senile dementia may be found to some extent in a proportion of well-preserved old people and that these changes increase with age.

(3) There also seems to be a 'threshold' effect. A plaque count of 11 and above per field separates most of those who had, during life, been demented from those who had been free from signs of mental deterioration. In Roth's example 90–100% of patients with functional psychiatric illness had 0–11 plaques per field while 85% of senile dements had 12 or more.

(4) The results are essentially similar with other morphological changes. When neurofibrillary changes, which cannot be counted precisely, were graded 'mild', 'moderate' or 'severe', subjects who received a

'severe' grading were almost entirely confined to the senile dementia group.

The other point that needs to be made is that histological changes tend to be present in all layers of the cortex in demented patients but tend to be restricted to the superficial layers in those subjects who have shown no significant intellectual decline.

ALZHEIMER'S DISEASE

Terry (1976) and Armbrustmacher (1979) have summarized the main histopathological features of Alzheimer's disease.

The brain size in Alzheimer's disease is shrunken in size, is strikingly atrophic, with diminished cortical and white matter and consequent enlarged lateral ventricles, and weighs about 1000 g on the average. This results in an abnormally large subarachnoid space. Atheromatous changes in the major vessels are not significant in most cases and are thought to be important in no more than 10–15% of cases.

The cortex is thinned and the atrophy diffuse though most severe in the frontal, temporal and occipital lobes. The meninges are often normal but may be diffusely thickened. Some of the cortical shrinkage may be related to loss of extracellular space.

The miscroscopic findings are characterized by widespread loss of neurones, with a mean decrease of about 55% and up to 70% gone from the deeper cortical layers. There is also – and this may be a cause of cortical thinning with important functional implications – reduction in dendrite arborization and a smaller than normal number of spines per unit of dendrite length.

There is a consistent appearance in the presentation of the pathological elements. These are made up of numerous senile plaques, neurofibrillary tangles, granulovacuolar degeneration and, occasionally, congophilic angiopathy.

As we have seen, *senile plaques* may be found in small numbers in about 70% of undemented old people over 65 years of age. In Alzheimer's disease the plaques are found throughout the cortex. They are easily stained with dyes such a Bielschowsky silver and are round and vary between 5 and 100 μm in size with a central dense core which contains amyloid. Surrounding this core is a crown of radiating, intensely argentophilic structures up to 5 μm in diameter. These are thought to contain the remains of degenerating mitochondria and numerous lamellar lysosomes, which seem to be derived from the mitochondria. Paired helical filaments are also found to be prominent in most plaques.

The mechanism that produces this degeneration is still a matter for conjecture but it would appear that the deposition of amyloid fibrils is the first event and the degeneration of presynaptic neurites (axonal endings) which provide the rest of the element is secondary. If the deposition of amyloid is indeed primary, an immunological process needs to be considered. It has also been suggested it may be due to a dying-back process due to viral, toxic or other process affecting the neurone. There seems also to be increased concentration of silicon within. The numerous mitochondria give it high oxidative activity and there is also an abnormal concentration of hydrolytic enzymes because of the many lysosomes.

As Terry has put it, any theory of the pathogenesis of the senile plaque must take into consideration the histochemical features of the lesion, its focal deposition, the restriction of the process essentially to cortical grey matter, the significance of the included structural elements and the relationship of this process to other pathological changes of senility. It must also be observed that the degenerating neurites might not necessarily be derived from cell bodies of neurones which contain the neurofibrillary tangles, since there are cases in which numerous senile plaques are seen with very few neurofibrillary tangles, and vice-versa.

The second major histopathological feature of Alzheimer's disease is the *neurofibrillary tangle*. The fibrillar components of the nerve cell body condense into twisted, convoluted masses in the cytoplasm. It is made up for the most part of highly stable paired helical filaments, each pair being about 20 nm at its widest and having a narrow twist about every 80 nm along its length. They are seen most readily in large neurones and are found in the greatest profusion in the hippocampus, amygdala, medial temporal lobes and frontal cortex.

The limbic system appears to be most profoundly affected but in the most severe cases the tangles can be found anywhere in the cortex. Subcortical grey matter, including the thalamus, basal ganglia and the cranial nuclei, is not typically involved.

Abnormal protein has been suggested as a cause of this change. If it is derived from normal protein, abnormal oxidation may be a factor. It is also thought that the high concentrations of aluminium demonstrated in senile brains might alter the assembly of conformation of normal protein. If the protein is abnormal, on the other hand, then either new genetic material introduced by either slow virus infection or genetic derepression would seem a feasible hypothesis.

The third histopathological change associated with Alzheimer's disease is *granulovacuolar degeneration*. This change is restricted to neurones in the cortex of the medial temporal lobe and consists of multiple vacuoles of $5-6$ μm in the cytoplasm of neurones. Each vacuole contains a single central $1-2$ μm granule. Clusters of vacuoles may cause the neurones to bulge and displace the nucleus.

This histopathological combination of cerebral atrophy with numerous senile plaques, neurofibrillary tangles and granulovacuolar degeneration with or without evidence of amyloid deposits in cerebral blood vessels (congophilic angiopathy) is characteristic of Alzheimer's disease.

Whereas this combination, when it is made up of the elements in substantial numbers, may be considered to be more or less specific for Alzheimer's disease, the same is not true for the individual elements. Neurofibrillary tangles have been described in the brains of boxers suffering from the 'punch-drunk' syndrome (dementia pugilistica) in the absence of senile plaques. This situation of tangles without plaques also obtains in the post-encephalitic form of Parkinson's disease and in progressive supranuclear palsy, in which a brain stem and diencephalic distribution of the tangles is also seen. It has also been reported in subacute sclerosing panencephalitis, as well as in the curious syndrome to be found among the Chamorros people of Guam where dementia is associated with parkinsonism and amyotrophic lateral sclerosis.

Plaques have been reported in Pick's disease, Creutzfeldt–Jakob disease and amyotrophic lateral sclerosis, while both plaques and tangles begin to occur in Down's syndrome in the third decade and are found in most cases surviving into the fourth decade and beyond. But the quantitative intensity of the changes, and the consistency of their combination, seem to be unique to Alzheimer's disease.

As will be discussed later, neurofibrillary tangles can be produced by aluminium when it is introduced into the cortex. Aluminium concentrations have been found to be elevated in a few patients with Alzheimer's disease. In rabbits lead intoxication can lead to neurofibrillary tangles. Plaques resembling human senile plaques have been produced in some strains of mice following inoculation with the scrapie agent.

Bowen (1981) has noted that senile plaques are often associated with capillaries, which suggests perhaps that neurones which are selectively affected may be vulnerable either because of their close proximity to an extraneural toxic factor (e.g. aluminium) or an infectious agent. Oxygen deprivation may be another factor for the pattern of hippocampal damage is similar in the hypoxic and the Alzheimer brain.

THE NEUROCHEMICAL BASIS TO THE PATHOLOGY

Thus histochemical changes to be found in dementia are complex and far from fully understood, let alone established. It would seem convenient at this stage to consider the neurochemistry of dementia in regard to the following

(1) cholinergic function;
(2) noradrenergic function;
(3) dopaminergic function;
(4) serotonergic function;
(5) hypothalamic function.

Bowen (1981) and Mann *et al.* (1982) have provided reviews of cholinergic dysfunction in relation to dementia.

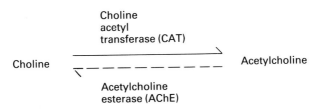

Figure 8.1   The production and breakdown of acetylcholine

Changes in cholinergic nerve cells were first reported in Alzheimer's disease in 1976, with reports of substantial losses of enzymes choline acetyl transferase (CAT) and acetylcholine esterase (AChE) (see Fig. 8.1). Since then these findings have been confirmed in both biopsy and autopsy brain tissue and the reduction in CAT activity has been correlated with the degree of histological change, the mental status of the patient and the severity of the dementia. This enzyme seems to be particularly reduced in the hippocampus.

A reduction has also been found in AChE activity in the brains of demented patients. However, there seems to be no significant difference in postsynaptic muscarinic cholinergic receptor concentration in the brains of age-matched subjects and those with Alzheimer's disease.

Quite apart from a reduction in the levels of the enzymes, the synthesis of acetylcholine, as Bowen has pointed out, is severely impaired in nerve endings from the cerebral cortex of patients with Alzheimer's disease.

The cholinergic system is apparently affected at an early stage in the pathogenesis of Alzheimer's disease for CAT activity is reduced in both biopsy specimens and port-mortem material from less severely impaired Alzheimer's disease patients. These observations – together with the relationship that has been noted between CAT activity, senile degeneration and the mental state – suggest that the depletion in cholinergic activity is of clinical significance. Further evidence for the early involvement of the cholinergic system comes from Perry (1979) who has shown that CAT activity is nearly halved as the plaque count rises from within to just beyond the 'normal' range with a less steep decline thereafter.

The enzyme may not be critical, however, in regulating acetylcholine synthesis, for at least in animal brains it is present in excess. Thus the data referring to a reduction in acetylcholine synthesis even in the presence of excess choline in Alzheimer's disease seem an important finding.

Smith and Swash (1978) postulated that damage to a cholinergic neuronal pathway running to or from the hippocampus might underlie the memory disorder which is the common presenting symptom of Alzheimer's disease. As evidence, they point to the fact that histologically the hippocampus is characteristically affected, CAT is depleted in the hippo-campus in the disorder, and that anticholinergic drugs administered to normal subjects can simulate some aspects of the memory defect seen in Alzheimer's disease.

While strong evidence exists for the presence of cholinergic defect, a belief in the sole or selective involvement of these pathways in Alzheimer's disease cannot be sustained. Cholinergic therapy has not demonstrated any consistent or long-lasting improvement in mental status following such treatment. This may only suggest that alteration in this kind of nerve cell may only be a part of a more widespread degenerative process. Further-more, as Bowen and Davison (1981) have pointed out, oral choline or lecithin would be unlikely to reverse the cholinergic defect for incubation media, and presumably the synapse in life, usually contain excess choline.

The greatest fall in cortical CAT is seen in the temporal cortex. There is evidence (Rossor et al., 1981) of reduction in CAT in amygdala and posterior hippocampus. They note that the disparity between the reduction in the posterior hippocampus and the anterior hippocampus is of interest, and may relate to previous reports that the posterior hippocampus shows more profound histological changes in Alzheimer's disease.

In Chapter 3 it was postulated that two forms of Alzheimer's disease, distinguished by course and outcome, may exist. The neuropathological and histochemical correlates of this clinical phenomenon are discussed at the end of this section.

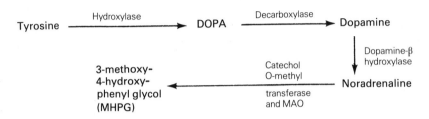

Figure 8.2   Synthesis and breakdown of noradrenaline

The noradrenaline concentration in brains from patients with Alzheimer's disease has been found to be lowered. It seems (Mann *et al.*, 1982) that deficiencies in the noradrenaline-containing nerve cells of the central nervous system may occur in Alzheimer's disease but not in dementia associated with cerebrovascular disease. The nerve cells they examined were melanin-pigmented cells of the *locus coeruleus* and the dorsal motor nucleus of the vagus nerve, on which this neurotransmitter system seems to be based principally. They found the number of melanin-containing nerve cells of the locus coeruleus and vagus nucleus is reduced in Alzheimer's disease by 60% with decrease of 22% in the protein synthetic capability of the remaining cells. These changes were matched by reductions in brain noradrenaline in eight regions, averaging 36%. In multi-infarct or vascular dementia, however, all of these features were unchanged, which led the authors to suggest that degeneration of the central noradrenergic nerve cells is a specific aspect of the pathogenic process underlying Alzheimer's disease.

Crow (1981) comes to a similar conclusion. He found the activity of the enzyme dopamine-β-hydroxylase (see Figure 8.2), which is a marker for noradrenaline-containing neurones, is significantly reduced in post-mortem brains of patients with Alzheimer's disease by comparison with control subjects or patients with multi-infarct dementia or depression.

As with CAT, a greater loss of nerve cells from the locus coeruleus seems to occur in those cases of Alzheimer's disease with high plaque counts and is correlated with the degree of mental impairment.

Discussing the inferences to be drawn from some of these findings, Mann *et al.* (1982) feel it is highly likely that atrophy and loss of the cells of the locus coeruleus and the dorsal motor vagus nucleus are responsible for the deficiencies in brain noradrenaline content, dopamine-β-hydroxylase activity and MHPG levels in brain and urine (see Figure 8.2) that have been demonstrated in cases of Alzheimer's disease. The non-pigmented cells of the vagus nucleus, which do not use noradrenaline as neurotransmitter, showed only slight loss of cells and only a modest reduction in protein synthetic capacity in their sample

As for the apparent preservation of the noradrenergic system in multi-infarct dementia, the same authors link this finding with the features of dementia which arise in multi-infarct dementia as a result of widespread tissue destruction rather than selective degeneration of specific nerve cell types.

A more recent report by Mann *et al.* (1984) considers the loss of neurones from the locus coeruleus as well as the nucleus basalis of Meynert (see later discussion) in patients with Alzheimer's disease of early and late onset. They have suggested that the extent of damage to the locus coeruleus is greater in younger patients than to the nucleus basalis whereas in older patients the damage is similar in both regions. They conclude that while disturbances in the cholinergic system may relate specifically to the impairment of cognitive functioning of Alzheimer's disease, it is possible that an especially severe degeneration of the noradrenergic system in younger patients is associated with the presence of certain of the neurological features discussed in Chapter 3.

Yates *et al.* (1979) have suggested there is no loss of dopaminergic neurones in Alzheimer's disease. Any apparent reduction in functional dopamine activity is attributed to a reduction in dopamine released by nerve stimulation rather than a reduced capacity of the tissue to store or synthesize dopamine. They have also considered the possibility that a reduction in physiological activity of the nigrostriatal dopamine system in Alzheimer's disease could be related to the loss of cholinergic activity indicated by the reduced levels of CAT in the caudate nucleus. They offer support from animal experiments that show that in the caudate nucleus, cholinergic dendrites may act presynaptically on dopamine-containing terminals to control dopamine release.

In passing, it appears that glutamate decarboxylase, which is a marker for gamma-amino butyric acid (GABA), is not related to either the intensity of histopathological change or mental test score in Alzheimer's disease (Bowen, 1981). This is confirmed by Perry and Perry (1982), who have shown that the level of GABA itself (together with the other amino acid transmitters glutamic and aspartic acids) is not significantly influenced by the number of plaques.

Bowen has also noted a reduction in the serotonergic markers, lysergic acid diethylamide (LSD) binding and 5-hydroxy indole acetate (5-HIAA) content, in the whole temporal lobe in Alzheimer's disease. CAT activity, but not LSD-binding, is reduced in less advanced Alzheimer's disease, which suggests that LSD-receptive cells degenerate after the cholinergic deficit occurs. Rossor (1981) has suggested that loss of 5-HT neurones is due to damage in the dorsal raphe nucleus and related areas. He believes this is further evidence of selective damage in Alzheimer's disease to certain groups of nerve cells whose ascending processes form part of the isodendritic core.

133

Bowen *et al.* (1983) have recently shown that biochemical markers of the 5-HT synapse are significantly reduced only in the neocortical tissue of pre-senile patients with histologically proven Alzheimer's disease.

Finally, the reduction in levels of arginine vasopressin (AVP) in certain regions of the brain in patients with Alzheimer's disease must be considered. Mann *et al.* (1981) have studied changes in nerve cell nuclear and nucleolar volume and cytoplasmic RNA which reflect alterations in polypeptide and protein production in the supra-optic and paraventricular nuclei. Significantly lower values of these indices had been found in Alzheimer's disease and cases of 'mixed' dementia when compared to controls, in the supra-optic and paraventricular nuclei. The authors point out that descending intra-cerebral pathways from these regions of the hypothalamus innervate, amongst other areas, the locus coeruleus and dorsal motor nucleus of the vagus. In turn, ascending adrenergic fibres from these latter regions seem to project to various parts of the hypothalamus. It has already been seen that adrenergic pathway dysfunction has been shown to occur in Alzheimer's disease but not in dementia associated with cerebrovascular disease, and the possibility of linking two regions of the brain through this finding must be a serious consideration. The changes in the ability to produce polypeptides in Alzheimer's disease are of importance in view of the interest being shown in the use of vasopressin and its analogues to improve memory deficiency. Perry and Perry (1982) examined the concentrations of different brain peptides in relation to the extent of the disease process in Alzheimer's disease and found that significant changes were confined to the more advanced cases and included reductions in cholecystokinin, somatostatin, neurotensin and increased substance P. The last trend was of particular interest as AChE is known to hydrolyse substance P.

Mann *et al.* (1982) have also speculated as to the mechanisms of action of these cell systems. They have suggested that the pigmented cells of the locus coeruleus and dorsal motor nucleus of the vagus, in conjunction with cells of the paraventricular and supra-optic nuclei of the hypothalamus, form pathways which act to maintain homeostasis within the central nervous system by regulating the rate of blood flow in the cerebral microcirculation and its permeability to water and metabolites through action on the capillary pericytes. They presume therefore that changes in functional integrity of these pathways of the *locus coeruleus* and hypothalamus in Alzheimer's disease may alter capillary permeability in such a way as to restrict local access of water or metabolites to the brain or prevent the removal of metabolic waste products with cytotoxic effects. Needless to say, all such explanations remain highly speculative at this stage.

THE NEUROPATHOLOGICAL CORRELATES OF POSSIBLE DISTINCTIVE FORMS OF ALZHEIMER'S DISEASE

The clinical distinction between two forms of Alzheimer's disease has been attempted in Chapter 3. The interesting histopathological and neuro-chemical correlates are considered here. It has to be said that while it has been customary to think of Alzheimer's disease as a cortical disorder, the evidence from histopathology and neurochemistry has been equivocal. Cortical atrophy is not invariable in Alzheimer's disease (Bowen, 1981). It is also known (Rossor *et al.*, 1982) that the cholinergic deficit in Alzheimer's disease, as assessed by CAT activity, seems not to affect all cholinergic systems or all the areas to the same extent and, in general, the earlier the age at death the more severe the cholinergic abnormality.

There seems to be a quite clear relationship between the site and level of CAT activity, histopathological abnormality and the severity of the clinical process in Alzheimer's disease. It was shown (Bowen *et al.*, 1981) that in the brain of demented patients suspected on clinical grounds of having had Alzheimer's disease but showing no histological evidence of senile de-generation, ACh synthesis was within the control range. Rossor *et al.* (1982) described cases of dementia with normal histology in which far fewer cortical areas showed significantly reduced CAT activity than in those with Alzheimer-type histology but with comparable involvement of the sub-stantia innominata. More recent attempts (Bird *et al.*, 1983) have gone further in comparing CAT levels between early-onset, more severe cases of Alzheimer's disease and late-onset, less severe cases. Several cortical areas had reduced CAT levels in the former but only the hippocampus was involved in the latter.

The origin of most of the cholinergic projections to the neocortex seems to be extrinsic, the cerebral cortex having few, if any, intrinsic cholinergic neurones. The substantia innominata is a subcortical structure which includes the nucleus basalis of Meynert and the nucleus of the diagonal band of Broca. It is part of what has been described (Rosser, 1981) as the isodendritic core, which seems to be the region containing the origin of cells which are initially afflicted in both Alzheimer's disease and Parkinson's disease. It is therefore possible that the origin of Alzheimer's disease, analogous to that of Parkinson's disease, is as a subcortical disorder. It is permissible, perhaps, to speculate that the less severe form of Alzheimer's disease obtains as long as the disease remains subcortical; when cortical structures are secondarily involved, the more severe form is seen. Cortical features are seen earlier in the course of the malignant form of Alzheimer's disease, found in younger patients with perhaps familial association, where the progressive stages of the disease, it might be argued, have telescoped.

When it is reported that cases exist of dementia running a clinical course similar to Alzheimer's disease, with cholinergic derangement but with no classical histopathological features to be seen, perhaps we ought to question our concept of Alzheimer's disease. Further work must, of course, be awaited but the notion of changing concepts and definitions is in keeping with the historical development of ideas regarding dementia and the underlying causative diseases (see Chapters 1 and 2). If this did come about it may also enable us to reconcile the difference of opinion that exists regarding the onset of dementia in Parkinson's disease (Chapter 3).

Rossor *et al.* (1984) analysed brains of patients with Alzheimer's disease, divided by age of death. They found that the older patients, dying in their ninth and tenth decades, had a relatively pure cholinergic deficit confined to temporal lobe and hippocampus, together with a reduced concentration of somatostatin confined to temporal cortex. By contrast, the younger patients, dying in their seventh and eighth decade, had a widespread and severe cholinergic deficit together with the abnormalities of noradrenaline, GABA and somatostatin. Their conclusion was that the results suggest that the 'young' cases of Alzheimer's disease represented a distinct form of pre-senile dementia which differed in important respects from the dementia of old age. Thus, the clinical, histopathological and neurochemical evidence in support of two distinctive forms of Alzheimer's disease appear to be strong.

VASCULAR (MULTI-INFARCT) DEMENTIA

Lishman (1978) has provided a description which is based on the work of Professor J. A. N. Corsellis.

The brain in vascular dementia may show localized or generalized atrophy, with thickened, adherent meninges. The ventricles are dilated and there may be cyst formation. There are scattered areas of infarction with areas of softening and scarring and sometimes an affected area of the hemisphere with a corresponding occluded vessel may be seen. The multiple infarcts involve the cerebral cortex as well as the internal capsule, the cerebellum, pons and the basal ganglia.

Vessels of all sizes are implicated. The main arteries at the base of the brain are thickened and tortuous with yellowish patches and nodular expansions on the walls. The lumina of the arteries are greatly reduced and may even be obliterated by thickening of the intima and subintimal plaques of atheromatous material. Small vessels within the brain substance may be thickened and show an 'onion-skin' appearance and occasionally the walls may be necrotic.

Microscopy reveals extensive loss and chromatolysis of the nerve cells, and the white matter may show irregular patches of demyelination. Scattered infarcts with cyst formation and reactive gliosis may be noted. Cystic softenings are said to be particularly common in the pons with microinfarcts in the hippocampi. Large areas of infarcted brain tissue showing necrotic degeneration with masses of phagocytes or, later, sclerosis with dense glial and fibrocytic infiltration may also be seen.

Roth (1980) has referred to a 'threshold' phenomenon for multi-infarct dementia analogous to the one proposed for senile dementia of the Alzheimer type. He has shown that below a figure of 50 ml of total infarction, dementia is rare; above it, dementia is almost invariable. It is also thought that the effects of infarction are potentiated by the presence of the senile form of change. With reference to previous studies he is able to show that senile change and softening each make independent contributions to the dementia, and their effects seem to be additive. Roth's point is that but for added brain damage caused by infarction, some individuals who might have had only senile changes may not have crossed the threshold into dementia.

Hypertension is well known to be associated with vascular dementia and Bowen and Davison (1981) have considered a possible mechanism. It seems the arteries of the brain respond to a persistent rise in luminal blood pressure by hypertrophy of the muscular medial coat with elongation of the arteries to produce a 'spiralling' effect. This increases with advancing age in arteries, arterioles, capillaries and venules throughout the whole thickness of the cerebral cortex and the white matter. The artery then becomes separated from the tissue by a fluid-filled channel and this results in a loss of sensitivity of the artery to changes in oxygen. Focal atheroma would accentuate and mask these changes, and any resulting infarction might lead to the 'threshold' being exceeded and to the occurrence of dementia. In animal experiments, ligation of the carotid artery leads to changes in the uptake and concentrations of some enzymes and soluble brain proteins.

The neurochemical changes noted in the vascular dementia are minimal and have been referred to in the previous section.

PICK'S DISEASE

A concise account is provided of the pathology of Pick's disease by Armbrustmacher (1979).

The brain, on naked-eye examination, shows severe, often discretely lobar, atrophy. The anterior portions of the frontal lobes are involved on both superior and inferior surfaces and temporal lobe atrophy is found involving the fusiform, inferior, middle and superior gyri, with a sparing of the posterior one-third of the superior temporal gyrus. When severe the atrophy is described as 'knife-edge' or 'walnut-like'. In some cases the atrophy as asymmetrical, with one side being more involved than the other. The lateral ventricles are dilated.

Microscopically, there is severe loss of cortical neurones, with gliosis, far more prominent than in Alzheimer's disease, extending into the white matter. Many of the neurones are swollen with chromatolysis. The hallmark of the condition, but not always found, is the Pick body. This occurs when neurones contain a discrete mass of argentophilic material in the cytoplasm, some 10–12 μm in size, which displaces the nucleus and causes swelling of the neurone. More commonly found are swollen neurones with pale cytoplasm. The inclusions are made up of neurofilaments and neurotubules and a preponderance of the former, which are more intensely argentophilic, gives the characteristic appearance of the Pick body. It has been postulated all these changes may arise as a reaction to an injury to the axon. Occasionally, neurofibrillary tangles, senile plaques and granulovacuolar degeneration may be seen.

HUNTINGTON'S CHOREA

The most severe and characteristic pathological lesion in Huntington's chorea is subcortical with marked atrophy of the caudate nucleus and the putamen. In most cases there is moderate to severe cerebral atrophy with the involvement of frontal and parietal lobes and a consequent dilatation of the ventricles.

The histological changes naturally correspond and there is extensive neuronal loss in the caudate nucleus and, to a lesser extent, in the other basal ganglia, thalamus, the brain stem and cerebellum. The cortical loss of cells follows the neuronal loss from the basal ganglia. With the loss of cells in the basal ganglia there is an extensive astrocytic reaction and spongiosis, The neurones which are left, often the larger neurones, have lipofuscin deposited in them.

The biochemistry of Huntington's chorea has excited interest and three neurotransmitters, gamma-amino butyric acid (GABA), dopamine and acetyl choline seem to be implicated.

In patients with Huntington's chorea the concentration of GABA, an inhibitory neurotransmitter, is reduced in the basal ganglia. Several groups of workers have reported a reduction in the level of glutamic acid decarboxylase, which is the enzyme catalysing the synthesis of GABA, in the same regions of the brain. GABA and glutamic acid decarboxylase levels in the frontal cortex and cortical CAT activity are normal. There are reports of reduction in the activity of choline acetyl transferase (CAT) and of muscarinic receptor binding activity in the hippocampal region.

Dopamine has been found in normal amounts in the caudate nucleus but its breakdown product in the cerebrospinal fluid, homovanillic acid (HVA), is reduced, which is taken to mean that less than a normal amount of dopamine might be undergoing breakdown to HVA.

It has been postulated that the chorea might be due to a deficiency of GABA or a relative overactivity of the dopamine. Workers have noted a relative sparing of the larger neurones in this condition. It may be (Armbrustmacher, 1979) that the lost smaller neurones might be internuncial cells with a presynaptic inhibitory function, and this might argue for a generalized lesion involving GABA neurotransmission.

Marsden (1982) feels the many other biochemical changes demonstrated in the choreic brain probably reflect neuronal loss. Thus substance P, angiotensin-converting enzyme and Met-enkephalin levels, all peptides which, like GABA, are thought to lie in strionigral and striopallidal neurones, are depleted in the basal ganglia. The functional significance of these abnormalities is said to be unknown.

A brief word regarding dementing Parkinson's disease may not be out of place here. Marsden (1982) has discussed the subject and has noted that while initial studies had suggested that CAT levels were unchanged, this may apply only to CAT activity in the striatum. [CAT activity in the frontal cortex and hippocampus of dementing Parkinsonian patients may be reduced.] The number of muscarinic cholinergic receptors also may be increased in some patients but remain normal in others. The Lewy body, the histological marker of Parkinson's disease to be found in the brains of all those afflicted, may be found in the substantia innominata and could thus be one of the links with Alzheimer's disease.

CREUTZFELDT–JAKOB DISEASE (CJD)

The pathological features of the disease in its usual and atypical forms have been discussed by Masters and Gajdusek (1982) and Armbrustmacher (1979).

The transmissible nature of CJD was established in 1968 and it was placed within the group of unconventional virus diseases which were the causes of scrapie (in sheep, goats and mink) and Kuru (an isolated disorder of human cerebellar ataxia in the eastern highlands of Papua-New Guinea).

Gross examination often reveals no detectable abnormality. However, microscopically, there may be a diffuse spongiform encephalopathy involving the grey matter of the cerebral cortex, the striatum, thalamus, globus pallidus, the nuclei of the cerebellum, mid brain, pons and medulla. The grey matter of the spinal cord may also be involved. The spongiform change consists of large numbers of vacuoles with an associated loss of cells and reactive astrocytic gliosis.

A distinction is drawn between the presence of fine vacuolation (spongiform change) which is characteristic of the disease and a non-specific change involving the coarse loosening of the brain parenchyma with severe gliosis (status spongiosus). Spongiform change is most severe and readily apparent in cases of 6 months' duration or less, whereas status spongiosus is seen in cases of longer duration. When spongiform change is well developed in the cerebral cortex, striatum, medial thalamus and the molecular layer of the cerebellum, the diagnosis of typical CJD becomes relatively easy.

No inflammatory cell infiltrate is found in either the meninges or the brain.

In Kuru, despite the absence of profound dementia, the cerebral cortex seems to be involved. Typical spongiform encephalopathy is found. There are also amyloid plaques (Kuru plaques) in more than 70% of cases of Kuru, especially in cases of long duration.

The amyotrophic form of CJD, which may have misled both Creutzfeldt and Jakob, is clinically and pathologically distinct from the transmissible spongiform encephalopathies in being untransmissible and is closer to amyotrophic lateral sclerosis. They show a loss of motor neurones in the spinal cord and brain stem, variable loss of pigmented neurones in the substantia nigra and a non-specific cortical neuronal loss and gliosis, especially in the fronto-temporal regions. There is no spongiform change.

There may be some pathological similarity between CJD and Alzheimer's disease, especially when the latter condition progresses rapidly with myoclonus. Plaque deposition may be found in both, and vacuolation is seen in some cases of Alzheimer's disease. However, all the evidence seems to suggest the conditions are nosologically distinct and there is little basis for thinking Alzheimer's disease might be transmissible in any way.

The fact that CJD is a transmissible disease with a postulated 'slow virus' agent which elicits no inflammatory reaction of the usual kind has led to the disease concept of 'slow virus' infection being considered in serious fashion. Armbrustmacher (1979) enumerates three main features of this disease concept.

(1) The diseases are caused by an infectious (transmissible) agent which has a long (months to years) latent period during which there are no symptoms of the disease.

(2) After the latent period, there begins a long, slowly progressive course of

symptoms due to the infection, with no remissions, almost always leading to a fatal termination.

(3) The disease is confined to a single species and to a single organ or tissue system within the species.

The proportion of case of CJD from which an isolation of virus can be made is more than 90%. Virus has been isolated from the cerebrospinal fluid, spinal cord, kidney, liver, lung, lymph node and blood. Peripheral routes of inoculation (intravenous, intramuscular, subcutaneous, intradermal and corneal) seem to be effective but the more peripheral the inoculation the more variable and longer the incubation period. The oral route of infection is effective for CJD, Kuru and scrapie.

Scrapie, CJD and Kuru viruses are resistant to inactivation by some of the methods used on more conventional viruses. However, scrapie virus is inactivated by autoclaving (121°C for 60 minutes) and by sodium hypochlorite (5% solution).

It is said (Masters and Gajdusek, 1982) the iatrogenic spread of CJD is the only mechanism that has been clearly demonstrated. It is, of course, a mechanism consistent with the presumed mode of transmission of Kuru, and one that is consistent with the biological behaviour of the CJD virus.

PRECAUTIONS WITH REGARD TO CJD MATERIAL

Great apprehension was expressed some years ago as to the dangers of infection that personnel dealing with patients, tissues or equipment infected with CJD might be exposed to. Masters and Gajdusek (1982) give comprehensive advice and instruction.

(1) There is no evidence in the natural history of CJD or Kuru for transmission by non-invasive bodily contact, though in view of familial incidence it remains a possible mechanism.
(2) No infectious virus has yet been demonstrated in tears, saliva, faeces, urine, sweat, skin or hair of CJD patients.
(3) There is no epidemiological evidence that medical personnel are at increased risk of developing CJD.
(4) The demonstration of infectious virus in the cerebrospinal fluid, blood and viscera means that appropriate precautions should be taken when handling this material, or when using instruments exposed to this material.
(5) The general nursing care of a patient with CJD poses no special problem, provided that open wounds are dealt with appropriately. There is no indication for isolation or 'barrier' nursing of patients. Linen and other materials in contact with open wounds or bed sores should be autoclaved or soaked in disinfecting solutions. Instruments (e.g. needles and syringes) which come into contact with blood, cerebrospinal fluid or other tissues should be disinfected or discarded by incineration, calling for no more than routine hospital practice.
(6) Laboratory personnel should take the same care as that exercised in handling blood, cerebrospinal fluid or other body fluids or specimens

taken from patients with hepatitis, tuberculosis, poliomyelitis and leprosy. Staff may be reassured that there is no recorded case of laboratory-acquired CJD infection.

(7) When surgery or brain biopsy is undertaken on CJD patients, the precautions consist primarily of attention to the adequate sterilization of instruments, usually by autoclaving. Instruments which cannot be autoclaved should be washed with sodium hypochlorite (5%) or phenol (10%). Care should be taken to avoid accidental self-inoculation with contaminated instruments.

(8) After fresh tissue is taken from the brain, cord and viscera for virological and other studies, specimens for histopathology can be fixed in 10% formalin to which phenol in a final concentration of 10% is added.

BRAIN CHANGES IN DOWN'S SYNDROME

The distinction between mental handicap and dementia was made and discussed in Chapters 1 and 2. However, a curious phenomenon, which has been known for several years but is assuming greater practical significance as patients with Down's syndrome survive into middle and old age, is the association between the syndrome and histopathological changes more usually found in Alzheimer's disease. Down's syndrome patients living into the forth decade and beyond almost invariably show senile plaques and neurofibrillary tangles.

It has been suggested that these patients have a reduction in the level of enzymes, choline acetyl transferase (CAT) and acetylcholine esterase (AChE). But there does not seem to be a reduction in level of activity of the brain noradrenergic system.

BRAIN BIOPSY IN DEMENTIA

Torack (1979) has listed three objectives in considering the need for brain biopsy.

(1) To obtain a biochemical assay of transmitters on the basis of the changes which have been discussed in previous sections.

(2) As a prognostic guide. A major criticism of brain biopsy is the high incidence of a normal biopsy. In 29 biopsies in demented patients Torack had 13 normal (45%) biopsies. But it was found that those patients with a normal biopsy had a much longer survival than patients in any diagnostic category. This may suggest that a normal biopsy affords a more favourable prognosis than any pathological category of dementia.

(3) To gain insight into pathogenesis, especially when the biopsy can be followed up later with an autopsy.

Torack believes a craniotomy and an open biopsy is the most desirable surgical procedure. The alternative is a needle biopsy when tissue can be obtained through a 14-gauge needle using suction aspiration. Frozen

141

specimens are quite valueless for diagnostic purposes in CJD but may be used in transmission studies.

IMMUNOLOGICAL ASPECTS

Behan and Behan (1979) have considered some immunological aspects of dementia and have summarized the evidence.

Some workers have postulated that the characteristics of ageing can be ascribed to a progressive failure of the immune system, particularly of thymus-derived, T cell functions. Others have suggested that impaired immunity in the aged represents genetic errors which occur as the organism ages, and that these are primary sources of immune dysfunction. Behan and Behan's summary of the evidence is as follows:

(1) Evidence now seems to suggest that amyloid in at least some cases is deposited in tissues under conditions of altered immunity. The incidence of amyloidosis rises progressively in old age and is accompanied by a loss of T cell function.
(2) Patients with Alzheimer's disease, when compared to age- and sex-matched controls, do have impaired T cell effects; the lymphocytes of these patients show a decreased ability to synthesize protein when stimulated by T cell mitogens at different concentrations.
(3) Antineuronal antibodies – found in immunological disorders where there is evidence of impaired T cell function – have been shown in Alzheimer's disease and can be detected in the elderly.
(4) The presence of oligoclonal bands in the cerebrospinal fluid of patients with Alzheimer's disease, which raises the possibility of an antigen inciting an immune reaction within the central nervous system.

OTHER METABOLIC CONSIDERATIONS

As Bowen and Davison (1981) have said, in normal ageing the quality of the nerve cell processes, rather than the number of neurones, declines with advancing age while in organic 'senile-type' dementia there is usually marked loss of neurones. In senile dementia the biochemical changes appear to be more extensive than might be predicted from histopathology, whereas in vascular dementia this does not seem to be the case. Thus, these authors feel, in senile dementia alteration in the metabolism of neurones may well precede slowly progressive changes in morphology. An early change in senile dementia, they feel, may be loss of sensitivity in the central mechanisms that regulate the response to changes in the requirement of the neurone for O_2 and nutrients.

Bowen and Davison have also considered some other pathogenetic factors. An endogenous gene defect may predispose individuals to Alzheimer's disease. A possible defect in transcription may be associated with a non-specific decrease in protein synthesis for there is yet no sign of an abnormal protein.

Another possibility considered is that a soluble toxic substance might be responsible for degenerative change; the evidence for this being that a heat-

142

labile high molecular weight factor has been found in extracts of Alzheimer's disease brains.

Yet another possibility must be considered in somewhat greater detail. Aluminium has been suspected as a neurotoxic agent (Crapper et al., 1978). They report that in Alzheimer's disease some brain regions have aluminium concentrations approaching 10–30 times the normal. In brains with neurofibrillary degeneration restricted to certain areas, elevated aluminium concentration was found in corresponding areas of the contralateral hemisphere. There was no such change in the brains of patients who exhibited multiple small infarcts without neurofibrillary degeneration but it has to be noted that aluminium has been described in certain other brain diseases – dialysis encephalopathy, the striatonigral syndrome (a variant of Parkinson's disease) and chronic alcoholism.

The normal function and the regulation of absorption and excretion of aluminium by humans are largely unknown. Crapper et al. (1978) believe the widespread but patchy distribution of aluminium over the cerebral hemisphere in Alzheimer's disease suggests a vascular route. The fact that brain aluminium is localized within the nucleus may simply mean the passive accumulation of aluminium by a failing cell.

Traces of aluminium may be found in the blood and the serum concentration is $19\pm6 \times 10^{-9}$ g/ml, though in the serum of patients undergoing renal dialysis for chronic renal failure it may be considerably higher.

Crapper et al. (1978) suggest that the brain uptake of the metal is not a simple overload phenomenon, and that aluminium accumulation in Alzheimer's disease is not accompanied by a general failure to exclude lead, iron, manganese, copper, zinc or cadmium.

Burnet (1981) has considered what he thinks might be a centrol role for zinc in the pathogenesis of dementia. It seems all or most of the enzymes concerned with DNA replication, repair and transcription – all of which require accurate transfer of information – are zinc metalloenzymes. The zinc atoms are intrinsic to the enzyme which loses its activity when the zinc is removed and may change its degree of 'error proneness' if the zinc is replaced. Burnet has suggested that this error proneness might lead to an inability to insert the zinc into newly synthesized enzymes which in turn leads to a 'cascading effect' resulting in dementia. The hypothesis remains entirely speculative.

Questions regarding the role of pigments and proteins in dementia have been raised by Mann and Yates (1982). They have argued that because accumulation of lipoprotein pigments with age can lead in some nerve cell types to decreases in protein synthetic capacity, it might be thought the extra reductions in Alzheimer's disease may be due to an excessive pigment accumulation. But as they themselves argue, there is little evidence to support this, and it is possible the presence of pigments in nerve cells in Alzheimer's disease indicates such cells to be old, but not necessarily diseased.

The same authors have considered the disruption in protein synthesis in Alzheimer's disease which is related primarily to alterations within the nerve cell nucleus. In the early stages production might be preserved even when the affected cells form and accumulate neurofibrillary material though, in later stages, when tangle accumulation may have surpassed a critical level, a deterioration in cell function is noted.

Mann and Yates, as noted before, have considered the effect of altered permeability of the microcirculation by a disturbance in the homeostatic mechanism. They feel that a widespread reduction in protein synthesis could be related to a more general metabolic disturbance, perhaps one arising from alterations in transport mechanisms which might conceivably prevent access to the brain of vital components, or allow the build-up within the brain of toxic substances.

SUMMARY

(1) The human brain increases in weight till the age of 18; the first significant decline in weight is around age 45 and weight loss is greatest after age 60. Loss of weight is greater in men than in women.

(2) There is a corresponding loss of neurones in parts of the cortex but the brain stem, apart from the locus coeruleus, is spared.

(3) There is an enlargement in ventricular size and alterations in the cerebral vasculature.

(4) Neurofibrillary tangles, senile plaques and granulovacuolar degeneration can all be found in the normal ageing brain; these may rise with age but they are never found in the profusion noted in Alzheimer's disease.

(5) Senile plaques can occur independently of neurofibrillary degeneration. There is a gradation in impaired mental status which correlates with the number of senile plaques.

(6) The *locus coeruleus* contains noradrenergic projections reaching the neocortex and its cells show a reduction in number with age with a corresponding decline in noradrenaline levels; the hypothalamus may show a fall in neurotransmitter levels as well as in choline acetyl transferase (CAT).

(7) There seems to be a highly significant correlation between indices of dementia as assessed by psychometric test scores and measurements of plaques, neurofibrillary change and granulovacuolar degeneration.

(8) A 'threshold effect' seems to exist; i.e. dementia is far more likely to occur once there are 12 or more plaques per field or 50 ml of infarcted tissue.

(9) In Alzheimer's disease the brain is shrunken in size and there is widespread cerebral atrophy and loss of neurones. There are also numerous senile plaques, neurofibrillary tangles, granulovacuolar degeneration and, occasionally, congophilic angiopathy. The impor-

tant feature is that these elements appear in combination and profusion.

(10) Neurofibrillary tangles have been described in 'punch-drunk' boxers, post-encephalitic parkinsonism, progressive supranuclear palsy, sub-acute sclerosing panencephalitis and in the parkinson-dementia syndrome of Guam.

(11) Senile plaques have been reported in Pick's disease, Creutzfeldt–Jakob disease and amyotrophic lateral sclerosis, while both plaques and tangles are found in patients with Down's syndrome when they survive beyond the third decade.

(12) In Alzheimer's disease there is a reduction in level of the enzymes, choline acetyl transferase (CAT) and acetylcholine esterase (AChE). These findings have been confirmed on biopsy and autopsy and have been correlated with the degree of histological change, the mental status of the patient and the severity of the dementia. The synthesis of acetylcholine is severely impaired in nerve endings and the involvement of the cholinergic system is thought to be an early feature of the illness. This deficiency has been related to changes in the hippocampus and defects of short-term memory.

(13) The noradrenaline concentration in Alzheimer's disease brain is lowered. This is not so in vascular dementia. There is a correlation with loss of nerve cells in the locus coeruleus and with high plaque counts and degree of mental impairment.

(14) There is also a reduction in level of 5-HT function, functional dopamine activity and in levels of arginine vasopressin (AVP) from the hypothalamus.

(15) In multi-infarct or vascular dementia there is localized or generalized atrophy, scattered areas of infarction, cyst formation and enlarged ventricles. The arteries are thickened and tortuous and their lumina may be obliterated.

(16) In Pick's disease there is often severe, discretely lobar, atrophy involving frontal and temporal lobes. The Pick body is characteristic but not always found.

(17) In Huntington's chorea the chief involvement is in the caudate nucleus and putamen. Cerebral atrophy is moderate to severe. A reduction in gamma-amino butyric acid has been noted.

(18) Creutzfeldt–Jakob disease, which is due to transmissible slow virus, is related to Kuru and scrapie, and shows characteristic spongiform change. There is no inflammatory infiltrate. A disease concept of 'slow virus' infection has been postulated.

(19) In view of the alarm that has been expressed about the dangers of the spread of Creutzfeldt–Jakob disease, a detailed account has been

given of the necessary precautions to be taken when handling patients, tissues or equipment.

(20) A brain biopsy may be essential for biochemical assay and useful in giving a prognosis or understanding pathogenesis.

(21) There is some evidence for an immunological basis to Alzheimer's disease.

(22) Excess aluminium and a functional deficiency of zinc have been suggested as factors in the pathogenesis of some dementias. The case is 'non-proven'.

(23) There is excessive lipo-pigment accumulation in Alzheimer's disease and also reduced protein synthesis. Whether they might have a role in the causation of dementia is unclear.

Further reading

(A full list of references is given at the end of the book)

Armbrustmacher, V.W. (1979). Pathology of dementia. *Pathol. Ann.*, **14** (11), 145-173

Bowen, D.M. and Davison, A.N. (1981). The neurochemistry of ageing and senile dementia. In Matthews, W.B. and Glaser, G.H. (eds). *Recent Advances in Clinical Neurology*. Vol. 3. (Edinburgh: Churchill Livingstone)

Masters, C.L. and Gajdusek, D.C. (1982). The spectrum of Creutzfeldt–Jakob disease and the virus-induced subacute spongiform encephalopathies. In Smith, W.T. and Cavanagh, J.B. (eds) *Recent Advances in Neuropathology*. Vol. 2. (London: Churchill Livingstone)

Roth, M. (1980). Senile dementia and its borderlands. In Cole, J.O. and Barrett, J.E. (eds). *Psychopathology in the Aged*. (New York: Raven Press)

Tomlinson, B.E. (1979). The ageing brain. In Smith, W.T. and Cavanagh, J.B. (eds). *Recent Advances in Neuropathology*. Vol. 1. (Edinburgh: Churchill Livingstone)

9
Management of the demented patient

As for the just cure, it must answer to the particular disease.

Francis Bacon (1561–1626)

If dementia is but the final common pathway of a number of conditions affecting the brain, it must be that the course of any one patient's illness will be determined by the pathology underlying the syndrome. While the prognosis may not invariably be hopeless – in the pre-senium anything up to 25% of all patients presenting with a picture of dementia may have treatable causes – it has to be conceded that at present all that can be anticipated in the majority of cases is an inexorable progression of the disease.

Thus 'therapy', 'cure' and 'rehabilitation' are unrealistic aims by the ordinary standards of medical practice and in those cases of dementia where reversal of the process cannot be countenanced it is quite unrealistic to expect patients to go back to leading the kind of life they did before they fell ill. Management of these cases is carried out with a far less ambitious aim in mind: to enable patients to live out their lives amidst their family and, if necessary, in a hospital with dignity and without too much distress to themselves or those around them.

However, a great deal, much of it of a simple nature and based on common sense and a knowledge of the resources available in the community, can be achieved and the management of the demented patient can in a limited way be a rewarding professional experience.

The form of general management applicable to all demented patients is considered first, and then an account of specific management of various dementias is given.

GENERAL PRINCIPLES OF MANAGEMENT

It will be clear from all that has been said in previous chapters that a diagnosis and formulation must be the starting point in any plan of

147

management. It is very likely – though we have no certain evidence available on the matter – that there is a time lapse between the onset of pathology and the appearance of clinical manifestations of dementia. This could be a matter of weeks, months or even years. This point is re-stated to emphasize there is no need for an unseemly rush into a diagnosis or to put an end to the collection of information about the patient or his illness. Every piece of relevant information has some bearing on the formulation, and every independent informant can assist in the process.

There is no question that the diagnosis of dementia is made by the clinician, and it will be he who will carry out or assess those investigations that may throw light on a cause of dementia. If a cause is found, its correction is likely to be engineered in the main by the same doctor or others to whom the patient might be referred. A case is often made for an initial assessment by a psycho-geriatric unit and there may be something to be said for a pooling of expertise. However, it will be understood that the majority of demented patients cannot be cured or even treated in strictly medical fashion, and while the diagnostic formulation is usually made in hospital, the overwhelming number of these patients will be managed in their own homes and in the community, by non-medical persons for the considerable part. It stands to reason therefore that the management of dementia must be considered from viewpoints other than the solely medical.

THE MULTIDISCIPLINARY TEAM AND THE DOCTOR'S ROLE

Even if a multidisciplinary force is given the task of managing the individual patient the doctor cannot abdicate his responsibility. Medical management cannot be a matter for committees. Quite apart from diagnosis, investigations and physical treatments, the doctor will have to take the legal, ethical and moral responsibility for the welfare of his patient. Some of these matters are discussed in the next chapter but it is sufficient for the present to emphasize that multidisciplinary management of the patient often entails greater rather than lesser responsibility on the part of the doctor.

Relationships within the multidisciplinary team, which may include district and community nurses, social workers, health visitors, occupational therapists, physiotherapists, speech therapists and volunteer workers, are a matter of some delicacy. Often the doctor is expected to be *primus inter pares* and yet this unofficial assumption of authority is then sometimes resented. A practical way to clear the air and avoid confrontation is to lay down the extent of each person's responsibilities and for team members to then desist from poaching or palming off jobs. Clearly the personalities of the participants count for a great deal, and if these can be brought into the open and acknowledged, so much the better for the functioning of the team.

Occasionally the doctor may be faced with an ethical dilemma concerning the patient *vis-à-vis* other team members who may well have different professional traditions and priorities. For instance, the doctor may feel the welfare of the demented patient is the paramount concern of the team, whereas the social worker, quite rightly, may be equally concerned about the disruption of family life which the patient's behaviour in the home might precipitate. There are no rights and wrongs in this kind of honest difference of opinion and it would be foolish to lay down fixed, inflexible rules. The doctor has recourse to one rule of thumb in these matters. Except in extreme cases – which are hardly likely to arise with demented patients and in any case will almost certainly be dealt with by the doctor in consultation with his colleagues and advice from professional bodies – the responsibility of the doctor is to the individual patient. The doctor–patient relationship, on these terms, has been enshrined in antiquity and the doctor, despite strong pressures to the contrary, might feel inclined to place this above family, social and community needs which might well be the major concern of a multidisciplinary team. In most instances, however, it will be obvious that matters need not reach this fevered pitch of principled confrontation if common sense is allowed to prevail.

INFORMING PATIENT AND FAMILY

Following the process of diagnosis and formulation the doctor is faced with several tasks. The first is to convey the information he has about the illness to the patient and the family. How much a patient and his family can be told without being unduly distressed or even, occasionally, devastated by the news is, of course, a matter of judgement. In the early stages patients are insightful and can, contrary to popular belief, grasp and make sense of what is happening to them. The general rule would be to be truthful and simple in explaining. Often the worry is about the immediate and more distant future, about pain, suffering, mental disturbance and, most of all, about being 'put away'. Most patients are reassured by being told that they can lead as normal a life as they can whilst being at home, though most relatives are considerably relieved that, if and when there is need, hospital admission can be arranged for shorter or longer periods. Complex discussions about the course of the illness and its management are best avoided in the average case lest they confuse the issue. Evasions, untruths and false optimism, even if kindly meant, have no place at all. Nature has a way of showing up false prophets and the last thing the patient needs at the start of a long and involved management of his condition is an undermined doctor–family relationship. The doctor will not go far wrong if he retails the known facts about dementia in a simple yet accurate manner.

THE ROLE OF THE GENERAL PRACTITIONER (GP)

Many of the issues mentioned in the foregoing paragraph are best tackled with the help of the GP. This stage is as good a time as any to involve the family doctor in an informal capacity in the management team. It would have been common courtesy in any case to have informed the GP of the results of the investigations and outcome. If the patient is to be managed at home, the first point of medical contact in any case of future emergency is likely to be the GP, and it pays to have him fully in the picture. For his part the GP, with his sometimes sounder knowledge of the family, may be able to explain matters further and perhaps more fully, and will also be able to provide the support the family often needs in those difficult early days.

ASSEMBLING THE TEAM

The multidisciplinary management team can be assembled with profit before the patient is discharged from hospital or outpatient department, wherever the investigations might have taken place. It is essential that all members of the team who are likely to have contact with the patient or his family be introduced to them at this meeting and any new members in the future be introduced by senior colleagues. In the nature of things most demented patients and their spouses are elderly, and any break in continuity that is implied in the appearance of new faces is a cause for alarm and anxiety. The team members should have met by themselves before the family is invited to meet the team and the outline of plans to be presented to the family discussed. Once the patient goes home the greatest danger is that he might be forgotten. It is bad practice to await crises before contact is renewed. At these times the patient and his family are seen necessarily at their worst and doctors and other staff, especially in a hospital setting, are too professionally busy coping with the problem in hand to pay attention to those apparently minor causes of anxiety which might mean a great deal to relatives. If there is a lurch from crisis to crisis the pressure for admission to an institution, even when it may not be strictly required, may grow to uncontainable proportions. Admission in these circumstances may well come to mean a permanent stay in an institution for a relatively well patient who could have been at home if his and his family's confidence had been sustained.

It is therefore important that contact be maintained at all times. How often and how intensive this contact must be will be decided by the resources of the Unit and the parts played by individual team members. The home help and the district nurse may have more frequent contact than other team members. If it is not possible for the whole team to see the patient and family at frequent intervals, a practical compromise would be for each team member to see them and report to others. The doctor then might see the patient once every six months, yet get an informed opinion regarding the patient and family far more often.

MANAGING AT HOME

The early stages of most dementias can be coped with by patients and their families without undue difficulty. Simple advice from the team about aids to daily living complement the common-sense steps families would take anyway. The capacity to adapt on the patient's part in the early stages, and the allowance families can make for patients, is usually impressive.

Formal behaviour therapy techniques are often used nowadays in institutional settings, and are discussed later, but their essentially simple principles can be adapted for use in the homes of demented patients with the co-operation of their families. At the simplest level the patient can be encouraged to keep a diary as an aid to memory. Reading a daily newspaper, preferably in instalments, watching television, listening to the radio, being reminded to look regularly at a watch, clock or calender that might be prominently placed in a room all help him with remembering current information that is so important to maintaining adult dignity. Encouraging the patient to remember, and to use a few familiar streets and to go shopping armed with a list, is another achievement that might gain worthwhile results. There is reason to believe, in an institutional setting admittedly but the point holds, that the most satisfying activities for demented patients at all stages of the illness are those of a domestic and social nature.

Relatives are often fearful that demented patients might harm themselves or their families and property by not paying due care and attention to gas or electrical appliances. Notice boards with large, coloured lettering, repetition of reminders, preferably with a demonstration of how it is done, can help patients to remember to use and turn off appliances and lock and unlock doors and windows.

Dressing, eating, toilet activites and attention to self-care and hygiene can be maintained by supervision and encouragement. The family may need to understand that slower and even relatively inefficient functioning is quite acceptable. The one thing demented patients are not short of is time, and this commodity can be put to good use if patience, understanding and tact are exercised by the attendants.

The doctor, whilst playing a part in advising on all these matters, can also ensure that patients' general health is otherwise sound, that he gets regular exercise and that he is sufficiently nourished and hydrated.

DAY CARE

What happens regularly to the patient during the day may be a critical factor in influencing his continued management at home. Most relatives are happy to look after patients in return for some life of their own. To a few it may be a need to go to work, to others just a pause in the daily grind. Demented patients, like all who are seriously and chronically sick, have the capacity to make intolerable demands on those who look after them and a respite is almost always welcomed. Day Hospitals and local authority Day Centres are two places which can offer a limited variety of activities and, more to the point, supervised care to demented patients. If the Day Hospital has links with the Unit in which the patient was originally assessed, and been looked after since, that would be ideal, but often new links have to be set up with a local Day Centre. The social worker can conduct these negotiations and an important requirement before admission to a Day Centre place is an undertaking from the recommending doctor that the patient's care will be taken over by the referring unit if his condition requires it. The team managing the patient should have no difficulty in meeting this reasonable condition.

TAPPING ALL FACILITIES

Quite apart from these supports, other sources of assistance are available from local authority bodies and voluntary organizations. An *attendance allowance* is available to relatives looking after a patient at home. Home helps can take the strain of domestic and housework off the shoulders of relatives and the provision of domestic laundry service is much appreciated by those looking after incontinent patients. The team social worker can advise on the range of services that patients and their relatives can claim, and she will keep abreast of all administrative regulations governing these locally.

HELPING THE HELPERS

In concentrating their energies on the patient the team must not lose sight of the difficulties of relatives, especially those of the spouse who is in most instances an elderly person. Support must be available to them on a regular basis. Some relatives carry a martyred air about them, but most ask for little more than gestures of appreciation and offers of support in this respect. It has already been shown that it is important to maintain their morale at all times and the acid test of a management team–family relationship is often a crisis. Most of these can be resolved in the home but in the event of significant illness or serious social or domestic upset the Unit must be prepared to admit the patient. An undertaking to this effect, given at the time of the first meeting and repeated as and when required, is very reassuring to relatives and there is nothing like a swiftly resolved crisis and a prompt return of the patient and family to the *status quo* to imbue relatives with even greater confidence in the team's competence and good intentions. Equally, there is nothing like crossed wires, uncertainty and dithering to destroy morale and trust. If teams of management can keep their word on these relatively straightforward matters the daunting problems of managing the demented patient will be eased considerably.

An organization which can offer valuable information and support to families is the Alzheimer Disease Society, 3rd Floor, Bank Building, Fulham Broadway, London SW6 (01–381–3177).

INTERVAL ADMISSION

If the patient is admitted for some emergency, the opportunity for an assessment of the dementia must be taken once the crisis is resolved. The extent of the investigations will once again depend on the resources of the Unit. The expectation in every case is that the patient will be returned to his home once his immediate medical difficulties have been resolved.

In the fortunate event of the patient leading a gratifyingly uneventful existence at home, the decision must be made about follow-up assessments being done without too much inconvenience to the patient. In the ideal situation all assessments and investigations can be done in the home or on an outpatient basis. Admission to hospital, indeed any change of environment, can cause great distress to patients, which in turn increases the danger of falsified test results.

THE TERMINAL ADMISSION

There is little real evidence that what precipitates admission of a patient to an institution, except in the kind of crisis discussed above, has much to do with any dramatic change in pathology or a sudden turn for the worse in his clinical state. On the other hand, the findings seem to suggest that admission is determined by social, domestic or environmental factors. A crucial reason may be illness, incapacity or death of the spouse. This is the reason why prognostication of inevitable institutional care is fraught with difficulty, being largely outside the doctor's province or his control.

The type of institution the patient ultimately goes to can vary, but once again there is little evidence that the institutions differ in the kind of patient they have as inmates or in the severity of their illness. They might be local-authority sponsored, warden-supervised residences or privately run nursing homes or a psychiatric hospital. Local availability and the financial status of the patient seem to be the more important determining factors in this regard.

Once patients reach an institution several other problems become apparent. Not only are they usually quite severely disabled by their illness but their social relationships might have broken down, for one or other reason, and often irretrievably. Then there is the matter of institutional life itself.

The problem of institutionalization is that on top of the disability due to the disease process *per se* there is an 'excess disability' as a direct result of the stultifying conditions of the environment. These include a lack of motivation on the part of the patient, a passive acceptance of his fate, loss of interest in his surroundings and an intellectual and emotional flattening. These are formidable obstacles to even the necessarily modest attempts at rehabilitating the demented patient.

However, a good deal of care can be provided. Attention to nutrition, hydration, self-care, mobilization and exercise are areas in which practical assistance can be provided to any patient. Constant endeavours must be made to interest the patient in his surroundings and keep him satisfyingly occupied. In this respect the activities available may not be materially different from those a devoted family might have achieved in the home, but the presence of trained staff is unquestionably a major advantage. It is important that the impression of a too clinical apprach to the patient and his problems is not conveyed to the relatives for their continued visits and links with the patient might well be what is best for him.

In an institution some attempt can be made to assess patients on an objective basis. The doctor and the psychologist will have their standardized tests but, as was shown in Chapter 4, there is advantage in combining these with ratings used by nursing and other staff. Many such scales are available but comprehensive ratings can be obtained with the Crichton Geriatric Behavioural Rating Scale (Robinson, 1961). The staff on the Unit might like to produce their own rating scale according to the needs of their patients and the staff resources available. The point is to establish a baseline for behaviour and then follow it up systematically. As with the Crichton Scale, the parameters could include mobility, orientation, communication, co-operation, restlessness, dressing, feeding, continence, sleep and mental state on a clearly defined, easily understood 1–5 scale.

As for other approaches to the general management of the demented patient, brief mention must be made of psychotherapy. Formal psycho-therapy of the traditional kind has been ruled out in most elderly subjects on theoretical and common-sense grounds and in the case of demented patients the question does not even arise. However, behaviour therapy might come to be seen in a very different light. It has been seen how the essentially simple principles of behaviour therapy can be applied in a practical way in the home by those looking after demented patients. In an institution more complex and detailed approaches based on the same principles can be attempted.

Lawton (1980) has considered the role of individual as well as group behaviour therapeutic approaches. It appears that in the limited number of instances in which individual behaviour therapy has been used in patients with organic brain disease, the patients, whilst being able to learn by contingent reinforcement, showed greater response to the reinforcement when it was continuous rather than when it was intermittent. It was also seen that discrimination among the different forms of reinforcers was difficult for the elderly patient.

'Milieu therapy' involves the use of elements in the therapeutic environment to reward desired activity in the patient. It seems when work done by patients was rewarded with cash they could be made to achieve more than by mere social rewards. In the 'token economy' desirable behaviours can be specified and rewarded by a generalized reinforcer, usually tokens, which can in turn 'buy' privileges or direct reinforcers such as food, clothing and sweets. In 'reality orientation' staff are trained to use natural conversational items of current information and orientation with patients, e.g. date, place, identity of people.

Whilst these approaches hold promise their effects on demented patients, as opposed to the elderly or the brain-damaged, has not been established and we shall have to wait and see. However, as Lawton (1980) has stated, while the results might be unclear in patients, an improvement has been noted in the attitudes of staff who have been formulating and carrying out these programmes.

SPECIFIC ISSUES IN THE MANAGEMENT OF THE DEMENTED PATIENT

The single dement

The assumption up to now has been that a demented patient will have a spouse or relative to provide care. This, of course, is not invariably so. Many elderly demented patients, mostly women, have to live by themselves. The need for regular, even daily, contact is even more urgent, and the vexed problem of weekend care, which is taken for granted when relatives are around, is a real one. There may be a tendency to give a higher priority to the dement living alone in allocating, say, a place at the Day Centre. Whilst this might seem sensible on the surface there is sometimes resentment on the part of relatives of other demented patients who might feel their efforts are not being appreciated or are being taken for granted. Once again these are not matters which can be sorted out by fixed rules but need the application of common sense and informed judgement. It will also be clear that the threshold for hospital admission will be lower for the patient who lives alone.

The agitated patient

The patient who is kept busy during the day in a satisfying variety of pursuits is the least likely to become agitated during the day or at night. Occasionally agitation may have a physical cause, illness or pain, and at other times it may be part of the syndrome. The use of psychotropic drugs in the elderly dement poses some special problems. To start with, these patients are smaller, their basal metabolism is lower, abnormally high blood levels may be reached because of both reduced degradation and diminished excretion; moreover, neurotransmitter levels often decrease with age so that neuroleptic as well as pyramidal side-effects dependent on transmitter levels may become more prominent; also, in Alzheimer's disease, functioning brain tissue levels may be reduced with a fall in number of receptor sites; many elderly dements suffer from somatic diseases which may make the prescription of psychotropic drugs more hazardous, e.g. in those with chronic bronchitis or those on anticoagulant medication; also paradoxical reactions are more common among the elderly, e.g. aggression caused by benzodiazepins (Van Praag, 1977; Reisberg *et al.*, 1980).

The following rules are usually recommended in psychotropic prescription for the elderly and are applicable to most dements.

(a) the initial dose must be small (one-third to one-half of the dose for a young adult and must be increased very gradually)
(b) the minimum effective dose should be established and constantly reviewed with the help of regular plasma or serum checks if possible;
(c) the minimum number of drugs, preferably one, must be used;
(d) the elimination of all unnecessary medication must be an even more constant endeavour than in the younger adult.

In the case of the agitated patient, popular belief has it that thioridazine (50–300 mg per day) is the neuroleptic of choice in the elderly. There is no consistent evidence for its superiority over others and it is possible that suitable titres of any established neuroleptic will be satisfactory. On the other hand, there may be something to be said for employing a drug in which the staff have confidence, whatever may be lacking in evidence.

It is also the usual experience that thioridazine in doses approaching the lower end of the given range is effective in dealing with milder forms of anxiety not amounting to agitation.

The choice of a sleeping draught for elderly patients is another vexed subject. The elderly require less sleep and in strictly medical terms may not require assistance with their sleep. A dement who is unable to sleep at home may get up, walk around and do whatever he wishes to without disturbing any one unduly, and being none the worse for this nocturnal activity. He clearly does not require a hypnotic drug though his relatives may need to be reassured. A patient behaving in identical fashion on a hospital ward can cause widespread disruption and circumstances are different. As with most matters in management, a reasonably satisfactory solution can be found if common sense is allowed to prevail.

The confused patient

A confusional state may well become superimposed on a dementia, and often constitutes a medical crisis for the patient and his attendants. As a rule a different pathology is involved and the commonest causes are respiratory, urinary or other infection, endocrine, metabolic or nutritional abnormality and, increasingly, medication, especially of the psychotropic kind. One can imagine a situation in which a patient becomes mildly agitated following a febrile infection, is liberally dosed with neuroleptics and hypnotics and ends up with an increasingly florid confusional state. The rational approach is the management of the underlying cause of the confusion.

Depression

As we have noted in previous chapters, depression may cause the clinical syndrome of dementia, be a symptom of the syndrome when its primary cause is some other pathology, or be found incidentally in a demented patient. In the present state of our knowledge the approach to the management of depression in each of these three instances is similar. Today, most cases of depression fortunately respond to antidepressant medication. The points made regarding neuroleptic medication are as applicable to antidepressant medication – an initial low dosage, divided into several daily doses, and a step-by-step increase in it. This works out as amitriptyline 10 mg t.d.s. with a cautious increase to the maximum tolerated by the patient. Dangers are visual disturbance, retention of urine, constipation, hypo-tension and confusion. Doxepin and dothiepin are advocated when there is any risk to the cardiovascular system and the quadricyclic drug mianserin may have less marked cholinergic side-effects.

If agitation is present with the depression, as often happens with the elderly, a sedative antidepressant such as amitriptyline may have to be used straight away, but in the exceptional case thioridazine may become necessary in addition to the antidepressant.

It is hard to find a place for the monoamine oxidase inhibitors in the management of depression in the elderly dement.

Fortunately, these days, the vast majority of depressive illnesses in and out of hospital have ceased to require dramatic intervention. Most cases of depression, whatever position they might occupy in the dementia syndrome, will respond to one or other of the drugs mentioned above. In the exceptional case leading to severe depression with psychomotor retardation, danger of inanition and risk to life, the question of electroconvulsive treatment (ECT) will always arise. However, unless it can be shown that the picture of dementia is due to depression alone there seems no justification for the use of ECT on a demented patient. Most dementias are a result of severe, chronic brain disease with a cardinal feature being memory involvement. Thus there would seem every reason to avoid further brain damage, an even greater assault on memory functioning and a more rapid progression of the dementia with ECT. What is usually required in the seemingly intractable case of depression is some patience with the drugs being employed, a rational outlook in changing from an allegedly ineffective drug (remembering it takes an antidepressant up to 2 or 3 weeks, perhaps longer in the elderly, to act, and noting that the cautious original dosage might have been only a fraction of what might be required for efficacy) to another and to redouble nursing effort to see the patient through without unnecessary trauma.

DRUGS FOR DEMENTIA

The idea of using a relatively simple chemical substance to correct the features of dementia has been, and must remain, a very attractive one. Several preparations, some now only of historical interest, have been employed and at one time or another claims, some cautious, some extravagant, have been made for almost every one of them. The truth, alas, is that there is not one of proven value in the management of any form of dementia.

The difficulties of assessment are manifold. The clinical syndrome of dementia may be common to all patients but almost nothing else is. Yet, populations of patients on whom the drugs have been tested have not usually been broken down according to definitive diagnoses. Furthermore, the distinction between such diverse groups of patients as 'organic brain syndrome', 'cerebral arteriosclerosis' and 'senile mental deterioration' has often not been made. Relatively few attempts have been made to consider severity of illness. Common sense informs us that the least severe cases must be the most promising for reversal of cognitive deficit. The difficulties of assessing memory, intellectual and personality functioning make cognitive testing an investigatory minefield, yet there are few objective psychometric tests in the reports. The criteria for a double-blind, placebo-controlled trial are not always satisfied and when it is known that a wide range of dosage may have varying effects on patients, with different optimal doses for different populations, few attempts have been made to test these. Finally, dementia is usually a chronic process and drug trials have necessarily to be continued for several months, if not years, for the effects of the preparations to become fully apparent. This has rarely been seen. Very often, too, it is not certain whether the drug really has a direct effect on the dementia or if it might be acting via an elevation of the mood state. The point, therefore, is that considerable scepticism is in order when assessing reports on these drugs, and only a handful which seem to have slightly greater promise than the rest are briefly mentioned in this account. A useful review is that by Reisberg *et al.* (1980).

Hydrergine

This is a preparation consisting of three hydrogenated alkaloids of ergot. Hughes *et al.* (1976) have reviewed 12 controlled studies involving the use of this drug over a period of 3 months. The variables which seemed to have shown significant improvement in patients given the drug were mental alertness, orientation, confusion, recent memory, depression, emotional lability, anxiety, fears, motivation, initiative, agitation, dizziness, vertigo, walking/mobility/locomotion, overall impression and global therapeutic change. These are impressive claims but the formidable methodological problems referred to in the preamble to this section, mainly as regards a lack of objective cognitive testing and a clear definition of diagnostic groups, remain. It has to be said that in a double-blind, placebo-controlled trial lasting 15 months, Kugler et al. (1978) showed that significant differences between hydrergine and placebo were not observed.

Cerebral vasodilators

These were first mooted for use in dementia on account of the belief that dementia was due to cerebral ischaemia caused by arteriosclerotic narrowing which might have been reversible. We now know this is unlikely to be so except in a minority of cases, and even then a consistent relationship between the behaviour of larger arteries whose narrowing is so reversed and the brain changes leading to dementia is not expected. However, a new rationale seems to have emerged for the testing of cerebral vasodilators. As was shown in Chapter 6, one of the distinctions between Alzheimer's disease and multi-infarct (vascular) dementia is in the preserved response to CO_2 stimulus in the former entity. CO_2 happens to be an endogenous vasodilatory stimulus, and a stimulus of a vasodilatory type introduced from outside was not unreasonably expected to lead to similar effects. However, whether vasodilation in practice can improve brain functioning by increasing blood supply and oxygenation remains to be seen.

Papaverine

Papaverine, an opium alkaloid without narcotic effect, is a smooth muscle relaxant which has been shown to increase cerebral blood flow, though it might be exerting some of its action by a dopamine receptor blocking effect (Branconnier and Cole, 1977b). As for its effects on dementia, the verdict must be 'non-proven'. The criticisms already made regarding drug trials in dementia seem applicable to many of the studies on papaverine. It seems possible that certain associated, but not necessarily related, laboratory changes, e.g. EEG features, might well be reversed (McQuillan et al., 1974; Branconnier and Cole, 1977a). Other vasodilators which have been investigated include cyclandelate and isoxsuprine. While individual mental symptoms have shown change, especially on less than rigorous objective testing of cognitive function, the place of these drugs in the therapy of any form of dementia can scarcely be said to be unequivocal.

A new substance, not related to any other drug currently being studied, is *piracetam*, which is a derivative of gamma-aminobutyric acid. It is thought to enhance associative cortical functioning and of interhemispheric transfer of information. In preliminary tests it has been shown to improve functioning in mild and moderate, but not severe, dementia.

An interesting departure, seemingly based on a rational understanding of biochemical deficiency, has been the use of choline-like substances. Acetylcholine (ACh) is synthesized from choline and acetyl coenzyme A (acetyl CoA) in a reaction catalysed by the enzyme choline acetyl transferase (CAT) and then broken down by acetylcholine esterase (AChE) as shown in this schematic representation.

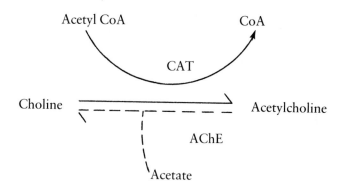

Bowen *et al.* (1976) had first suggested that the activity of CAT, the enzyme that catalyses the conversion of choline to acetylcholine, was selectively reduced in the brains of patients with Alzheimer's disease. A reduction in CAT levels and activity may indicate presynaptic cholinergic damage, and leads to decreased acetylcholine synthesis and release. Since postsynaptic muscarinic receptors seem to be preserved it is likely that attempts to increase acetylcholine synthesis and release, or to stimulate these post-synaptic receptor sites directly, might modify some clinical aspects of Alzheimer's disease if cholinergic neurones were involved in its patho-physiology. CAT activity is also reduced in brains of patients with Huntington's chorea. Unlike in Alzheimer's disease, however, muscarinic receptor sites are also reduced and cholinergic therapy has not suppressed chorea in these patients (Growdon and Corkin, 1980).

The results of pharmacological experiments indicate that cholinergic neurones can influence learning and memory function. Physostigmine, a centrally active AChE inhibitor, elevates ACh content and thereby stimulates postsynaptic cholinergic receptors by slowing the breakdown of ACh released by the presynaptic neurones. The clinical features noted have included improvement in long-term memory storage and retrieval and reversal in scopolamine-induced memory deficits. But physostigmine, which has very short-lived actions, has to be given by injection while direct-acting cholinergic agonists may be given orally but have serious muscarinic side-effects.

Food contains little free choline and most exists in the form of lecithin, which has been shown to increase brain ACh levels in animals. As most patients are said to prefer lecithin, which is tasteless and free of the fishy odour associated with choline, it seemed natural to use this in some of the trials.

159

In the investigation of demented patients, memory deficit has been the feature chiefly studied, partly because disturbance of memory is a common early feature of Alzheimer's disease and partly because of an apparent link between cholinergic mechanisms and learning and memory. Growdon and Corkin (1980) have reviewed seven studies published between 1977 and 1979. The number of patients in these studies ranged from one to ten and only one study dealt exclusively with mild cases of Alzheimer's disease (Signoret et al., 1978). Significantly, this was the only trial to produce even modestly encouraging results. The workers administered 9 g of choline chloride daily to eight patients, subjected them to cognitive testing and found that three of their patients in the pre-senile subgroup showed slight improvement in delayed recall and delayed learning. As the other six series were even less striking in outcome, one can understand that at present the role of choline-like substances in reversing the symptoms of dementia is far from established.

Vascular dementia

In the present state of knowledge this term must necessarily embrace cases of dementia due to diverse varieties of arterial disease. The general principles of management of the dementia are the same but the higher incidence of focal lesions make more specialized demands on physiotherapists and speech therapists.

Vascular dementias must ultimately derive from brain lesions but the relationship of these lesions to those produced by the common strokes is not clear. As Mohr (1978) has pointed out, while 34% of strokes may be associated with large-artery athero-thrombosis, lacunar infarctions, which we have good reason to incriminate in the causation of vascular dementia, cause only 19% of strokes. If, therefore, the prevention of strokes seems an eminently sensible way of reducing the incidence of vascular dementia, one must appreciate that different mechanisms may operate in the causation of the different variety of strokes.

The three areas which might be thought at present to hold the greatest promise in reducing the incidence of strokes are:

(a) the control of hypertension;
(b) the management of transient ischaemic attacks (TIAs);
(c) the management of certain cardiac conditions.

Control of blood pressure elevation is thought to be the single most effective means of stroke prevention, and prevention of stroke recurrence also rests on effective antihypertensive treatment (Wolf and Kannel, 1982). While this point is now generally acknowledged, a word of caution must be sounded. Clinicians, who are well aware of the danger of sudden and substantial reduction in blood pressure, have also to keep in mind, as was hinted in Chapter 6, that an elevated blood pressure might well be keeping up a faltering supply of blood to the brain and any precipitate or marked reduction in pressure raises the possibility of disturbance to an adaptive phenomenon.

Although only 10% of strokes are preceded by TIAs, and in case of lacunar infarctions the incidence is even rarer, this is a group of patients who are thought amenable to intervention in the practice of cerebrovascular disease. The risk of stroke following TIA is highest in the first few months, falls off after that and may be up to 10 times that in the normal population (Mohr, 1978). Apart from control of hypertension, there is now a case for the use of aspirin, especially in the male patient, in doses of up to 1200 mg daily. A case for a smaller dose exists (Marcus, 1977) and the actual dose would reflect the current state of cardiological opinion. Its effects are thought due to a reduction in a platelet-induced hypercoagulable state, though curiously the therapeutic effect is noted only in men. The place of anticoagulant medication has always been the subject of controversy but it is believed some modest claims can be made for warfarin sodium. Whisnant (1977) and Walsh *et al.* (1978) could report favourable results. The customary strictures on patient tolerance and physician vigilance apply.

Strokes are associated in about 15% of cases with atheromatous disease in surgically accessible parts of the carotid artery system. Extracranial vascular surgery for patients with strokes has been available from the 1950s and is of proven value in stroke prevention, though of little or no value in the developing or completed stroke. A number of workers have commented on the improvement in 'mental state' following carotid endarterectomy even in cases of completed stroke, but it will be quite clear that the fully established dementia syndrome is a far cry from subjectively reported and uncritically noted 'mental' symptoms. The crucial criticism is, however, the difficulty in establishing a relationship between surgery conducted in the territory of the large arteries which are affected by atheromatous disease and the lesions that give rise to dementia of vascular origin.

Cardiac causes of strokes include post-operative complications following insertion of a prosthetic valve (reduced by anticoagulant therapy), atrial myxoma, aortic valvular disease, chronic left ventricular failure and the cardiomyopathies. The reduced incidence of rheumatic heart disease and subacute bacterial endocarditis is reflected in the lower incidence of strokes due to these conditions.

The other risk factors for stroke which it might be rational to control in those who have, or might be at risk of developing, vascular dementia are diabetes mellitus, hyperlipidaemia and heavy cigarette smoking.

Huntington's chorea

Apart from the management of dementia on the lines outlined there is a special need to consider the peculiarly distressing features of this condition. Suicide, self-mutilation, alcoholism, criminal behaviour, domestic violence, promiscuity and sexual deviation are not uncommon features and there is a high incidence of childhood death in apparently disease-free individuals (Oliver, 1970). There is a case for the provision of services run by individuals with a special interest in the disease in those localities with known concentrations of cases, but for the time being the doctor must rely on the work of the excellent voluntary Association to Combat Huntington's Chorea (COMBAT). Its addresses are:

National office: Borough House, 34a Station Road, Hinckley, Leicestershire LE10 1AP (Telephone: 0455–615558).
London office: 108 Battersea High Street, London SW11 3HP (Telephone: 01–223–7000).

It is recommended that patients and all those looking after them be put in touch with COMBAT as soon as the 'disease' is diagnosed so to avail themselves of the many services that are provided.

In addition, the control of choreiform movements becomes necessary. Phenothiazines, especially thiopropazate (in doses of up to 40 mg daily), have been used with success. Tetrabenazine (up to 100 mg daily) and haloperidol (up to 15 mg daily) also have their advocates. The mode of action, whether it might be a direct effect on the involuntary movement by a restrictive rigidity or merely secondary to the control of psychosis and tension, is unclear. Stereotactic surgery has been mooted, especially when chorea is more disabling than dementia in young patients, but there is a real risk of aggravating the dementia.

Following reports of disordered gamma-aminobutyric acid (GABA) metabolism, isoniazid, an anti-tuberculous drug which acts as an inhibitor of GABA amino-transferase, the first enzyme-degrading GABA, has interested some workers. It has been shown to elevate brain GABA in animals and when it was given in high doses – with serious risk of liver damage – to a small group of patients there was improvement in mood and chorea (Perry et al., 1979). But in the absence of controlled trials, its efficacy and safety remain to be proved.

Computer-held regional genetic registers could help to reduce the chances of a diagnosis being missed and families being needlessly exposed to the distress that a condition such as Huntington's chorea can cause.

At present the only effective means of limiting the disease is for 'at-risk' individuals – the disease is due to an autosomal dominant gene – to remain childless. The risk is not always 50% but varies with age. COMBAT has assessed the risk to offspring as follows:

Risk at birth   = 50%
     at 10 years = 50%
     at 20 years = 49%
     at 30 years = 44%
     at 40 years = 33%
     at 50 years = 12%
     at 60 years = 2%
     at 70 years = 0%

The risk to the grandchild of a choreic, where the child's parent is symptom-free, is generally about half of the parent's risk (or, more accurately, the product of the age-related risks). For example, if a symptom-free patient had a risk of 33% at the age of 40 years, his or her child aged 20 years would have a risk of $49 \times 33 = 16\%$.

Whilst these rough-and-ready guides are adequate for most ordinary situations, the counsel of a Genetic Advisory Centre is strongly advised in every case.

Knowledge of the risks and the facts are not usually sufficient. Prospective parents are still faced with a difficult choice and even when alternatives such as adoption, sterilization and artificial insemination are offered may decide to accept the risk outlined to them. This brings us into the realm of ethics but it cannot be considered a failure of genetic counselling whose purpose is to alert and explain to individuals the hazards in a particular situation rather than to force them into exercising an unwilling choice.

Tyler (1979), in a study in South Wales, found families of patients were largely ignorant of the illness, only a third of them having received any information. The children, in their turn, were more exposed to information but a third of them had nevertheless produced yet another generation at risk.

The ability to identify healthy carriers might provide an impetus to attempts at preventing the disease. Earlier attempts with EEG recordings, studies of abnormal movements in various parts of the body, measurement of GABA in the cerebrospinal fluid, cell membrane investigations, CT screening and genetic linkage studies have all drawn a blank. But recent studies on the behaviour of skin fibroblasts in culture (Spokes, 1978) and the response of 'at risk' subjects to L-DOPA – which produces excess dopamine which it is thought might induce choreiform movements before the onset of the disease – hold a certain promise. These procedures will raise ethical questions and will be taken up in the next chapter.

Another procedure which will bring greater certainty whilst raising ethical questions of another kind is pre-natal screening. Some attempts have been made in this direction but it is very early days yet.

Other specific dementias

Treatment for dementias due to endocrine and metabolic causes is the correction of the underlying condition. In hypothyroidism, thyroid replacement therapy generally results in rapid and significant improvement in cognitive function. The failure of some patients to make a recovery appears to be related to the duration of the hypothyroid state. It has been suggested that no patient with dementia due to hypothyroidism of more than 2 years' duration makes a completely successful recovery.

Most patients with dementia due to hypoparathyroidism have been reported to recover their cognitive capacities with treatment. As with other 'secondary' dementias, early diagnosis would appear to be important to full recovery.

When vitamin B_{12} deficiency has developed sufficiently to involve disorder of higher functions, replacement therapy brings about more swift and complete improvement in the haematological state and in the peripheral neuropathy than in the dementia.

In general paresis, penicillin in the form of intramuscular procain penicillin in a total minimum dose of 6 million units is now the treatment of choice. Apart from a risk of the well-known 'Herxheimer reaction', the treatment is straightforward and the cerebrospinal fluid, once it has been cleared, is checked every few months and then annually. Treatment must be restarted if abnormal cellular elements reappear in the cerebrospinal fluid. All other treatments of general paresis are of historical interest only.

A major problem in the management of idiopathic normal pressure hydrocephalus (NPH) is the relatively low percentage of patients who have been reported to respond favourably to neurosurgical intervention (Katzman, 1978). The usual treatment for NPH has been the shunting of cerebrospinal fluid through a tube running from the ventricles through the jugular vein into the atrium of the heart, the so-called ventriculo-atrial shunt. Success rates have varied from less than 10% to 86%. Katzman (1977) reported that, on the average, 64.7% of patients with secondary NPH responded favourably, whereas in the idiopathic form only 40.9% did so. The incidence of mortality following shunts may be 6–9% and the incidence of various shunt-related complications up to 40%. The most serious complication is formation of a subdural haematoma, but meningitis and embolism have also been reported. Blocked shunts are a problem, especially when they are ventricular in origin. A lumbar–peritoneal shunt, being without valves and placed at a distance from the brain, may cause few problems.

Amantidine was held to be of some value in Creutzfeldt–Jakob disease, more through a metabolic or biochemical action than by a direct antiviral effect. Confirmation as regards its efficacy is still lacking. The question of the prevention of Creutzfeldt–Jakob disease belongs more properly to pathology and has been taken up in Chapter 8.

SUMMARY

(1) The majority of dementias are progressive and irreversible but selected groups of patients, e.g. the pre-senile, may have a substantial number which might be treatable.

(2) The aim of management in most cases of dementia is to enable patients to live out their lives in dignity and without unnecessary suffering to themselves or their families.

(3) A firm diagnosis and a full formulation by the doctor is the starting point in the management, but a multidisciplinary task force will be required to look after the patient and his family.

(4) Whilst the diagnosis is made in the hospital, the vast majority of demented patients are looked after in their homes. The multidisciplinary team can meet patient and family in the hospital and follow up the care in the home.

(5) It is important that regular contact be established and maintained with the patient and family even if further admission to hospital does not occur. The GP may also have a useful role to play.

(6) In the early stages patients often adapt to their disability and families make allowance for failing functions.

164

(7) If the patient is given ample time and encouraged to do what he can, if he is allowed to move about in familiar surroundings, if instructions can be repeated and stated in another mode, he will make a better adjustment to his disability.

(8) Attendance at a day facility helps the patient and relieves the family of the burdens of care for a few, regular hours each day.

(9) It is important that the managing team be aware of all the facilities and services patients are entitled to.

(10) The family, which might be under considerable strain, must be supported at all times.

(11) Voluntary organizations play an important role in the care of patients in the community and provide considerable support for the families. The addresses and telephone numbers of organizations dealing with Alzheimer's disease and Huntington's chorea are given.

(12) Patients may have to be admitted to hospital in cases of acute medical or social crises. Vigorous intervention at this stage may restore the *status quo*.

(13) There is little evidence that the reason for the final admission to hospital is medical. On the other hand the loss of a spouse may be one important factor.

(14) A problem in institutions is the danger of 'excess disability'. Sensible, practical activity geared to the patient's abilities and needs guards against this.

(15) Continued objective assessment of the patient by the various professionals is of assistance.

(16) Though formal psychotherapy is of little or no use, simple behavioural approaches may have a place.

(17) Most demented patients, being elderly, have special problems with drug therapy. Doses need to be smaller and more closely monitored than in the younger patient.

(18) Thioridazine (up to 300 mg daily) is of value in the agitated patient; amitriptyline in small doses (beginning with 30 mg daily) may suffice for depression. There is no place for MAO inhibitors or ECT in the demented patient.

(19) Confusion in the dement may be due to injudicious psychotropic medication. When due to infection or metabolic cause the treatment is of the underlying condition.

(20) Several drugs have been used in a direct attempt to reverse the symptoms of dementia. None has been proved to be of consistent value and the methodological problems in their assessment have been serious.

(21)Though ordinary strokes may not usually be associated with those cerebrovascular lesions causing dementia, a common-sense approach would be to reduce the incidence of all strokes and vascular insults. The steps to take are to control hypertension, manage transient ischaemic attacks and certain cardiac conditions, and the control of diabetes mellitus, hyperlipidaemia and excessive cigarette smoking.

(22)Huntington's chorea patients may cause considerable distress to their families who require a great deal of support. Drugs are available for the control of choreiform movements. Genetic counselling is a vital measure in the prevention of the illness.

(23)Successful treatment of most of the 'secondary' dementias due to endocrine, metabolic or vitamin disorders depends on early diagnosis and a prompt commencement of therapy.

Further reading

(A full list of references is given at the end of the book)

COMBAT (1982). *Huntington's Chorea*. A booklet for family doctors and other professionals. (Association to Combat Huntington's Chorea)
Office of Health Economics (1980). *Huntington's Chorea*. (London)
Reisberg, B., Ferris, S.H. and Gershon, S. (1980). Pharmacotherapy of senile dementia. In Cole, J.D. and Barrett, J.B. (eds). *Psychopathology in the Aged*. (New York: Raven Press)

10
Dementia: epidemiological, social, legal and ethical considerations

> One touch of nature makes the whole world kin . . .
> William Shakespeare (1564-1616)
> *Troilus and Cressida*, III, iii, 165

> the government are very keen on amassing statistics – they collect them, add them, raise them to the nth power, take the cube root and prepare wonderful diagrams. But what you must never forget is that every one of these figures comes in the first instance from the . . . village watchman, who puts down what he damn pleases.
> Sir Josiah Stamp (1929)
> (quoted by Schoenberg, 1978)

EPIDEMIOLOGY

In 1960, Kay *et al.* (published 1964) undertook a survey of the prevalence of mental illness in the aged in Newcastle. Their objectives also included the ascertainment of the kind of care the elderly mentally ill were receiving, especially as regards the proportions being cared for in institutions and in their homes. These workers found that around 10% of the population over the age of 65 had dementia of some kind, and that in half these cases, or 5% of the population, the condition of the dementia could be termed severe.

Kay *et al.* (1970) repeated the survey with somewhat greater rigour to exclude the more doubtful cases and also derived age-specific rates for senile and multi-infarct dementia (Tables 10.1 and 10.2).

Table 10.1 gives the prevalence of organic brain syndromes, broken down by sex and age. Table 10.2 gives the sex differential prevalence in the two main types of dementia, with a breakdown by age. Kay *et al.* (1970) also showed a steady increase in prevalence of dementia till the age of about 80 and a rapid acceleration of rates beyond that age. They suggested that rates for males and females were not significantly different, the apparently higher prevalence among females being presumably due to their ability to survive old age better.

167

Table 10.1 Prevalence of organic brain syndromes by age and sex (after the Report of the Royal College of Physicians, 1981 from Nielson, 1962; Kay *et al.*, 1970 and Kaneko, 1969)

Age (years)	Males		Females		Both sexes
	Percentage	SE of percentage	Percentage	SE of percentage	Percentage
65–	*3.9	± 0.97	*0.5	± 0.35	2.1
70–	4.1	± 1.21	2.7	± 0.85	3.3
75–	8.0	± 1.99	7.9	± 1.67	8.0
80+	*13.2	± 2.64	*20.9	± 2.68	17.7
All ages	6.2	± 0.76	6.3	± 0.68	6.3

SE = Standard error
* = Difference between males and females statistically significant ($p<0.01$)

Table 10.2 Sex differential prevalence in dementia (after Roth, 1978)

Patients	Senile dementia (%)		Multi-infarct dementia (%)	
	65–74 years	75+ years	65–74 years	75+ years
Men	1.7	4.4	3.4	6.7
Women	4.1	9.3	1.1	2.3

The prevalence of pre-senile (i.e. under 65) dementia is in general about a tenth of that for senile dementia. There is a gradual increase after this age is passed, and then a more rapid increase. By the age of 85 a third of a population may be designated as having senile dementia. Beyond this age there is a tendency for the rates to level off.

Figures from around the world are comparable as Table 10.3, which gives the prevalence of chronic brain syndromes over the age of 65, shows.

Table 10.3 Prevalence of mild and moderate or severe chronic brain syndromes in patients aged over 65 (after Kay, 1972 and Report of the Royal College of Physicians, 1981)

	Percentage moderate or severe dementia	Percentage mild, if known
Kay *et al.* (1964), England	5.6	5.7
Kay *et al.* (1970), England	6.2	2.6
Syracuse study (1961), USA	6.8	–
Nielson (1962), Denmark	5.9	15.4
Kaneko (1969), Japan	7.1	52.7
Hagnell (1970), Sweden	9.1	7.0

The Office of Health Economics (1979) has made a series of projections for the number of demented patients in England and Wales according to population trends. On the basis of the overall prevalence rate of 10% among the population aged 65 years and over they estimated that some 715 000 people in England and Wales were affected by dementia at the end of the 1970s. By 1990 it is thought there might be 7.6 million persons over the age of 65 – contributing 760 000 cases of dementia – and then a small fall, to about 727 000 cases, by the year 2000.

168

In the United States, where the number of dements is estimated to be between 1.5 and 2 million, Eisdorfer and Keckich (1980) believe the proportion of elderly persons will grow to 29 million or 12% of the US population by the end of this century, and will continue to increase until at least the year 2020, when approximately 18–20% of the population will, it is thought, be 65 or older.

As for the population aged 80 years and over in England and Wales, amongst whom there is a prevalence of over 20%, it has been estimated that the number of affected individuals will increase by over 41% to a total of 388 000 over the same period of time (about 20 years) that cases among those aged 65–69 are projected to fall by 17% (OHE, 1979). It is therefore clear that it is the change in age structure of the elderly population, rather than its overall size, that will be a major factor in determining the numbers of demented patients.

It can also be seen that many of these projections will be in serious error if the natural history of dementing conditions or the structure of populations changed in significant ways. It has been suggested that the onset of senile dementia, presumably of the common Alzheimer variety, is now delayed. This may alter the numbers of dements, as would a dramatic further improvement in life expectancy. In this regard some concern has been expressed that a comprehensive epidemiological study on the Newcastle lines has not been carried out for 20 years.

The *incidence* of dementia has been less conclusively worked out. Kay (1962) had suggested the annual average incidence of senile psychosis might be 2%, and Bergmann *et al.* (1971) make an estimate of annual average incidence of 1.4%. Estimates of incidence rates vary widely, the chief discrepancy being between those studies, as those mentioned, based on random sampling and psychiatric and personal interviewing which produce an incidence rate of 1.5% per annum and those based on newly reported (case register) cases with rates around 0.5% per annum (Report of the Royal College of Physicians, 1981).

The value of epidemiology does not lie simply in providing us with figures to help health planning. Some epidemiological findings may turn out to be of aetiological importance. The unusual age- and sex-related rates of prevalence of some dementias may imply a heterogeneity of the disease process. This is an area on which epidemiological research might throw some light. On the other hand, while there is no epidemiological evidence for the incrimination of purely social factors as poverty and isolation in the onset or progression of most dementias, the role of environmental factors has been duly noted with regard to general paresis and Creutzfeldt–Jakob disease. A contribution from epidemiology to unravelling the part played by metallic toxins, trace metals, atypical infections and other environmental agents is awaited.

Multi-infarct or vascular dementia has been variously estimated to contribute between 10% and 20% of all dementias. Age- and sex-related rate differences are clearly discernible and allowance has to be made for the particular composition of a population under study. Even allowing for this, there is reason to believe the incidence of vascular dementia has been overestimated in the past and workers nowadays tend to be conscious of this.

It is believed that the prevalence of manifest Huntington's chorea normally ranges from between 4 and 7 per 100 000 of the population but, as Table 10.4 shows, there can be considerably greater rates in various geographical pockets. The figure of 7 per 100 000 would give 4000 active sufferers in the United Kingdom, though COMBAT, the Association to Combat Huntington's Chorea, believes that the figure might be nearer 6000. It has also been suggested that there has been a recent increase in the numbers of individuals carrying the gene as a result of increased fertility in affected individuals. Increased libido associated with a decrease in inhi bition and personal responsibility has been suggested as being contributory.

Table 10.4 Prevalence of Huntington's chorea (from Office of Health Economics, 1980)

Country	Area	Authors	Year	Prevalence per 100 000
England	Northampton	Oliver	1970	7.5
	Bedfordshire	Heathfield and McKenzie	1971	7.5
	East Anglia	Caro	1977	9.4
Scotland	SW Scotland	Bolt	1970	5.6
	Moray Firth	Lyon	1962	560*
USA	Rochester, Minnesota	Kurland	1968	6.7
South America	Venezuela	Negrette	1970	2000*
Australia	Tasmania	Brothers	1949	17.4
	Victoria	Brothers	1964	14.8
Japan	Aichi	Kishimoto	1959	0.4

* Very small populations studied

The prevalence of Creutzfeldt–Jakob disease, given its protean presentation, is often difficult to detect in community surveys but Marsden and Harrison (1972) found 3 cases out of 84 demented pre-senile patients (3.6%) in a hospital investigation. The disease has a world-wide distribution and has been documented in more than 50 countries. Masters and Gajdusek (1982) claim to have recorded more than 2000 cases world-wide, and give 0.43 deaths per million as having been the average annual mortality in the US in 1978. They have noted a steadily increasing trend since 1970 and attribute it to increased awareness in physicians. Several foci have been identified in Czechoslovakia, Italy, Hungary and Israel and a very high incidence of the disease in Libyan-born Israeli Jews (more than 30 per million) is referred to by these authors.

Pick's disease is often difficult to distinguish from Alzheimer's disease with any confidence on clinical grounds, and the attempt is not usually made in surveys of pre-senile dements. Katzman (1978) believes the incidence of idiopathic normal pressure hydrocephalus among patients with pre-senile dementia is between 5% and 6%. The incidence of this condition among senile dements is only about 0.2% (Jellinger, 1976). General paresis, which used to fill the wards of mental hospitals in the last century, is now a rare illness. Dewhurst (1969) studied the records of patients admitted to six mental hospitals between 1950 and 1965 and found 91 cases.

SOCIAL ISSUES

In England and Wales today there are more than 700 000 dements, i.e. 10% of the population aged 65 years and over. Half of this number may be expected to be severely demented.

For every one of these demented patients being looked after in an institution there are five living in the community. On this basis it had been estimated that at the end of the last decade in England and Wales there were probably about 600 000 elderly people suffering from varying degrees of dementia living at home (OHE, 1979).

Those patients in the community live alone or are looked after by their relatives. Institutional care is provided in psychiatric and geriatric hospitals, local authority residences and private nursing homes. One-third of the elderly demented population in institutional care are to be found in residential homes. The official Department of Health and Social Security guideline for elderly severely mentally infirm patients is a recommended 2.5–3.0 beds being made available for every 1000 of the population and a similar provision in addition is made for elderly severely mentally infirm day patients. The actual provision is considerably smaller and in the case of inpatients the future projection is for a fall in number of places.

The question of the range, variety and suitability of institutional care is a very complex, and at times controversial, one and has been dealt with in great and impressive detail in the publication by the Office of Health Economics (1979). As far as the individual doctor is concerned, however, he is in practice quite powerless to make fundamental assumptions regarding the provision of institutional care. The construction and closure of hospitals and homes hardly come within the province of the average doctor. The most he can try to achieve, probably, is to inform himself of the issues in a general way, try to influence the powers-that-be by reasoned argument, and get on with the management of the patient and helping the family. The doctor, the patient and the family constitute much of the society of the demented patient and it is to social issues which have a bearing on that society that we must now direct our attention.

Demographic trends, as we have seen, suggest that the problem of dementia will become even more serious for the rest of this century. The elderly have already begun to form an increasingly large proportion of the population. Table 10.5 shows the rough structure of the relevant population over the past eight decades and gives a projection for the beginning of the next century. For 1978 these figures worked out to 3.1 million men aged over 65 years and 6.4 million women over 60 years. The table also shows that the proportion of the population over 75 years has increased rather faster than the elderly as a whole. It is expected that the proportion of very

171

elderly people in the population will continue to rise, at least until the early 21st century.

Table 10.5   The elderly as percentages of the total population (after Blane, 1982)

	1901	1931	1978	2001
Over retirement age	6.3	9.8	17.0	16.0
Over 75 years of age	1.3	2.2	5.2	6.1

The proportion of women among the elderly rises rapidly. Women already make up 70% of those over 75, and 80% of those over 85 years of age. As we have seen before, it is the structure of the very old population that is likely to influence the numbers of demented patients in the population. As some 20% or more of the population aged over 80 years is likely to become demented, it is estimated this would mean an extra 100 000 patients in England and Wales by the end of this century.

Most demented patients and their spouses, like children under 15 years of age, come under what has been called the 'dependent' section of the community and have to be supported by the 'productive' sector which is aged between 16 and 64 in present-day society. Given current trends in employment, it is quite likely this range will be narrowed even more, and the burden of supporting the dependent members of the community will fall on even fewer shoulders. In unvarnished practical terms this must mean increased taxation if services are to be kept at the present, barely adequate levels, not to mention any attempt to improve them.

Much has been made of the virtues of managing the demented patient in the community, with a substantial part of the care being taken over by the families of the patients. Families in modern society tend to be 'nuclear' with, in the usual instance, a man and a woman, both of whom are likely to be at work to provide for a couple of dependent children. These families also tend to be mobile, moving in search of work, education for the children and to improve their style of life. The enormous social changes that we have seen in recent times have had as their effect the release of the individual to seek greater personal freedom, and the inevitable concomitant of this has been a loosening of bonds, especially between generations. It is not easy to see how an elderly dement, who has become dependent on two counts, can be fitted into this setting of the modern nuclear family in the absence of serious, regressive change back to the society and values of some generations ago.

The moral question of whether a family should be expected, in a civilized modern society, to care for patients who have a serious medical illness is taken up in the final section of this chapter and the cost to a family, where it can be measured, will also occupy us in a while. But the point about availability of family members to look after the elderly sick can now be considered. The spouse apart – and, given the differential rates for life expectancy, many very old women are destined to widowhood – the number of persons available in the family of the demented patient has fallen. The average family in Victorian England had seven children; within a century this number has fallen to fewer than two. Furthermore, divorce and widowhood have meant a greater prevalence of one-parent families.

Traditionally, an unmarried daughter staying at home provided the care needed. Today, that person is likely to be married, have a family of her own and be at work. In 1901 there were 13 single women aged between 45 and 60 to look after 100 elderly persons; now there are only 5 (Locker, 1982).

It would therefore be a facile assumption that, given present trends, the average family can provide care over a period of time to seriously and chronically ill persons. It has been shown (Sainsbury and Grad, 1966) that a community-based service of provision to the mentally ill is effective in reducing the frequency of admission to institutions but is only achieved at the expense of imposing a considerable burden on the family.

The financial cost to the community is a very real one. Millard (1981) estimated that at £150 a week, and with the assumption of 2 years of life after admission, the cost of institutional care for a patient would be £15 000 per head. Rising costs must already (1983) have put this figure at least £2000 out of date.

The OHE (1979), assuming that one-quarter of the resources consumed by elderly patients can be associated with dementia, estimated that for 1976–1977 the management of dementia cost about £300 million, yet no account could be taken of the cost of other hospital expenditure, the use of drugs and, of course, the financial burdens experienced by caring relatives.

The OHE also refers to a study by Opit (1977) into the costs of domiciliary support for patients receiving home nursing services. It was shown that services for a patient receiving weekly 4 hours' visiting, 4 hours of home help and two meals cost the equivalent of non-medical resources given to a person in a residential home and about two-thirds of those available to individuals in an established geriatric inpatient unit. Opit has further claimed that 5–10% of all patients would cost more to support at home than in hospital or residential care.

Any attempt to quantify the value of services and care provided by relatives cannot be a serious undertaking yet the effects on the family – in terms of sacrificed careers, the leisure activities given up, the cost of neglect to the children in the family, the stresses and strain, both psychological and physical – can well be imagined.

However, the reality is that five out of six demented patients are looked after in their homes, and it would be of interest to know the factors that determine this mode of care. Bergmann et al. (1978) could show that of patients living in the community while being day patients at a hospital, some 70% would die or be placed in institutional care before the end of 12 months since they were identified by the research team. The most important factor affecting the patient's continued existence in the community was family support: 46% of those patients who had children were still able to be at home at the end of 12 months. Patients who lived with a spouse were more vulnerable, while those who were at the greatest risk were those patients who lived alone.

As for the future, concern naturally has been expressed about the sufficiency of services for the large numbers of demented patients. While the adequacy of services in absolute terms is rightly a matter for concern, a continuing worry must be the extent to which patients and their families have even now an awareness of the nature of dementia and of the services available. There is little doubt that considerable ignorance exists regarding the mental problems of the aged. The OHE publication quotes work which has shown the extent of lack of knowledge among members of the primary care team and points to the relative neglect of the elderly by social workers among whom apparently it is usual to assign untrained and junior members to elderly patients. As with any issue that has a social component, it must be expected that it will be attitudes that will determine the care the dement will receive.

The whole approach to the management of the demented is likely to be coloured by the attitudes to the elderly in general. As their proportions in the population grow the elderly will become more visible. They happen to be weak, dependent and obviously different in appearance; they are among the poorest members of the community and they tend to live in its most deprived parts; they may be rigidly conservative in outlook and cling to their own 'culture' – which will place a nostalgic emphasis on 'wholesome-ness' and a disdain for the new, the avant-garde and for nonconformism generally – which is likely to exert an effect on the culture of the younger members of the community; above all, they will clamour for services and they have votes as well. It does not require an exceptional feat of imagination to grasp that the aged may well become another disadvantaged minority. Already the term 'ageism' has been coined to denote those attitudes and acts of bias against the elderly and any reading of human history must show that such an anticipation of another class of victims of bigotry is not altogether fanciful. Since everyone everywhere who survives grows old there will be an almost unique prospect of universal prejudice. *Almost*, because women, often as a disadvantaged majority, have been there first.

Quite apart from attitudes to the elderly, the question that must be raised is how much those who can provide will do so. Public expenditure and taxation are usually portrayed as matters of economic and political concern. Ultimately, of course, providing for the sick and those disadvantaged in general is a moral concern which springs from a desire to help those who are less fortunate. The portents for generosity in this direction are not good, and widespread cutbacks in social welfare are not only in the offing but the climate of moral and political opinion seems to favour it increasingly. In a democracy, the government, by and large, does the urging of those in the majority or at least those representing the largest number of voters. If what makes political sense is to cut back expenditure on services to the elderly, so it will be. The rather tragic irony seems to be that the aged, psychologically inclined to political conservatism and averse to expenditure on welfare services, may well be urging political decision-making to their own disadvantage.

If greater individual – meaning patient as well as his family – responsibility is going to be required in the future what private contri-butions can be made has to be considered. The total cost cannot be worked out with any measure of accuracy but it would seem unrealistic to expect the patient and his family to bear more than a fraction of the cost in a private capacity. The cost of investigation of the dementia and the management in home and hospital with the full panoply of doctors, nurses, social workers, various ancillary therapists, and laboratory technicians, not to mention the cost of equipment, must surely be beyond the means of the vast majority of the ordinary population, let alone the aged living on their pensions. As for private health insurance schemes, these have traditionally been reluctant to finance long-term management of geriatric and psychiatric illness. The prospects for privately financed research into dementia on anything approaching the scale that will be required are also remote. No reasonable alternative can therefore be envisaged to providing adequate, humane care other than a state-financed system of care for the demented patient.

As we have implied, in a democratic society, political will is determined by the moral outlook of the ordinary, individual voter and in this capacity we must seek whatever comfort we can.

LEGAL ASPECTS

The legal issues which have a special bearing upon dementia may be looked at from two angles. On the one hand we have to consider the involvement of the demented patient in criminal activity; on the other, the provisions made by law to protect the patients and his property have to be appreciated in the total management of the demented patient's condition. Even if some of these matters are dealt with primarily by lawyers, the doctor, who is a permanent professional member of the team managing the patient's illness, needs to have a knowledge of the principles underlying the legal issues, and may indeed have to draw the attention of the family and the other members of the management team to these.

Most demented patients, being elderly, will very rarely commit offences. Moreover, chronic brain syndromes have never featured as important causes of crime in any major survey of offences due to the mentally abnormal offender. An occasional presenting feature of dementia can, however, be some criminal activity which might have resulted as the product of loss of judgement and of inhibitions, and is most likely to be seen in patients with Huntington's chorea and Pick's disease.

Walker (1968) has discussed the possible reasons for an abnormal criminal's conduct and some of his points may be modified to apply to the demented patient.

(1) Low (meaning lowered) intelligence may prevent him from understanding that the nature of his act was wrong.
(2) A disorder of mind may distort his ethical views, or intensify normal impulses to a degree which makes it difficult or impossible for a person even with normal self-control to resist them.
(3) The disorder may lead him to underestimate the seriousness with which his crime is regarded at law, or it may lead him into situations in which even the mentally normal person may be vulnerable and tempted to commit an offence.

175

(4) His disorder may simply mislead him into thinking he will not be caught.

The type of criminal behaviour does not usually extend beyond such minor offences as shoplifting and exhibitionism. Incidentally, the dirty old men of popular belief and imagination are not usually demented or mentally ill in any formal sense. They are socially and sexually inadequate persons who have grown older into even further social and sexual isolation.

It is also possible that some of the features associated with dementia, most especially depression, might facilitate the commission of serious crimes. Depression means not only the condition which gives rise to what some workers have been pleased to call the 'dementia syndrome of depression' but also the mental state in which acts of violence are possible. Depression occurs most frequently in the early stages of dementia when the integrity of the brain is presumably largely preserved and it is possible for a dementing patient to plan and commit a serious crime. The place of depression in violent criminal behaviour, especially in the culture of England and Wales, is well attested to. Presumed depressive murder followed by suicide of the aggressor occurred over a period of years in a third of all murder suspects in England and Wales (West, 1965).

Criminal responsibility

As all dements are over 14 years of age they are subject to the strictures of the criminal law. The law presumes that every person accused of a crime is sane and responsible for his actions until the contrary can be proved and the burden of proof rests with the defendant.

Three questions need to be determined.

1. Fitness to plead

This is with regard to the ability to plead at the time of the trial. When medical evidence as regards the unfitness of the accused to plead is presented, he may be compulsorily detained in hospital without limitation of time. In instances of recovery, clearly not applicable to the majority of cases of dementia, the accused may be brought back for trial.

2. Responsibility

Impaired responsibility was a concept brought into effect in English law by the Homicide Act of 1957 to deal with those instances when factors other than 'disease of reason', which might have a bearing on an accused person's actions at the time of the alleged crime, could be taken into account.

Section 2 of the Homicide Act sets out the following:

'Where a person kills or is party to the killing of another, he shall not be convicted of murder if he was suffering from such abnormality of mind (whether arising from a condition of arrested or retarded development of mind or any inherent causes or induced by disease or injury) as substantially impaired his mental responsibility for his acts and omissions in doing or so being a party to the killing'.

The result of this Act is that the question of responsibility, or lack of it, need no longer depend on academic arguments about the nature of madness and whether or not a loss of reason was involved. The effect of a successful plea is to reduce the charge from murder to manslaughter, and so open up the options of disposal.

3. Not guilty by reason of insanity

This historic defence on the grounds of insanity stemmed from the McNaghten Rules of 1843, but following the Homicide act of 1957 and its provisions for dealing with diminished reponsibility is a rarely heard plea.

The manifestations of dementia come under the meaning of the term 'mental disorder' for the purposes of the Mental Health (England and Wales) Act, 1959, consolidated by the Mental Health (Amendment) Act of 1982, and the Mental Health (Scotland) Act, 1960.

The sections relating to the compulsory admission to hospitals of patients are as applicable to cases of dementia as they are for patients with functional psychiatric illness. These are sections 25, 26, 29 and 30, the 'court order' sections of 60 and 65 and sections 72 and 73 providing for compulsory admission of convicted persons to psychiatric hospitals as allowed by the England and Wales Act.

In addition, section 135 of the England and Wales Act provides for a Mental Welfare Officer to obtain a warrant authorizing a constable to enter premises in order to remove a mentally disordered person to a hospital (or a place of safety). This order expires after 72 hours.

Section 136 of the same Act allows a constable who finds a mentally disordered person in need of immediate care and control in a public place to remove him to a place of safety, usually a psychiatric hospital. This order too expires after 72 hours.

A rarely used further safeguard – or infringement of liberty, depending on one's point of view – for old rather than chronically sick people living in squalor and neglect is section 47 of the National Assistance Act of 1948. The community physician can apply to the local authority for the compulsory removal of such persons to an institution. A magistrate has to support the order. The institution, which must indicate a willingness to accept such a person, and the person concerned, must normally be given a week's notice and the order is effective for a period of 3 months. In an emergency the National Assistance (Amendment) Act of 1951 can be invoked and this notice need not be given, but the order then lasts only for 3 weeks.

Testamentary capacity

Demented patients are usually at the time of life when wills need to be drawn up. The law requires that a person making a will has a 'sound disposing mind' and the doctor may find himself involved in a case in which a challenge is mounted against the provisions of a will on grounds of the testator's alleged unsoundness of mind. The doctor may be required to assess the patient's mind with regard to the following questions:

(1) Does the patient understand the nature of the act of making a will and its effects?
(2) Does the patient know the nature and extent of his property?
(3) Does he know which persons have a claim on his property?
(4) Can he form a judgement on the strengths of the claims made by these persons on his property?
(5) Has the patient expressed himself clearly and without ambiguity? The will need not be made in writing and gestures and nods made by the patient to questions put to him by an authorized person are in order.

The assessment by the doctor is with regard not to will-making in general but to the will in question, and clearly circumstances will be different with simple and complex wills and mild and severe cases of dementia. The doctor is usually advised to examine the patient alone, to take note of any undue influence that might be exerted on the patient and to make and preserve verbatim notes. It is important to assess the effects not only of illness but also of any drugs that might have been administered to the patient. Finally, as doctors are sometimes called upon to witness wills, it is important to realize that if he is a witness as well as a beneficiary the will becomes void.

The Mental Health (England and Wales) Act of 1959 provides for the management of the property and affairs of patients by a Court of Protection. When satisfactory medical evidence can be given to the Court of Protection that the patient by reason of mental disorder is incapable of managing his property, the Court appoints a Receiver. Three Medical and a Legal Lord Chancellor's Visitors ensure the affairs of the patient are being properly conducted.

SOME ETHICAL ISSUES

It is possible to direct attention to only a few of the many ethical issues which have a bearing on the clinical practice of, and research into, dementia. These ethical issues may have to be put in the balance against a condition which is often malignant and afflicts over 700 000 individuals in the United Kingdom and up to 2 million in the United States, reducing life expectancy by between one-third and one-half. Yet, we have seen that in patients under 65 years of age there may be anything up to a 1 in 4 possibility of detecting a treatable cause of dementia. Whatever might be the cause of a dementia, any hope of reversing the changes due to pathology probably rests on an attack on the earliest manifestations of the condition. Moreover, it is reasonable to assume, there will be little prospect of any available drug or chemical currently undergoing investigation being established in a scientifically acceptable way unless diagnostic categories in the dementias are established and respected. To test a potential therapeutic agent against a heterogeneous class of clinically diagnosed dementia and to expect results is equivalent to exhibiting undifferentiated fevers to a new antibiotic. It would be as unacceptable and futile a practice with regard to dementia as it would be in the rest of clinical medicine.

Approaches to both these issues, establishing the early as well as the precise diagnosis of a dementia, may involve a recourse to biopsy of one or more regions of the brain and thus brings an ethical dimension to the problem. A few of the technical aspects of brain biopsies are dealt with in the chapter on pathology but it can be said here that, as with all operative procedures, there is a small but definite risk. More important perhaps than the actual medical risk is the emotion surrounding this invasion of the last great human anatomical unknown. Quite apart from fears of physical assault on what is still presumed by many people to be the seat of the soul and personality there is probably the nagging suspicion that technicians who get that far into relatively unexplored territory may, in their determinedly amoral fashion, go further by experimenting with and manipulating patients. A concerted programme of health education might go some way towards educating doctors and the general public in a general way, but ultimately it is the individual demented patient and his family who need to take decisions about bits of his body.

In the early stages of a dementing illness the patient possesses a relative measure of insight and may be able to give informed consent as to a biopsy or other invasive procedure and to any therapeutic intervention that might follow the investigation. The trouble arises when dements progress from this to a state in which many functions, including reason, judgement and insight are all gradually lost. Some drugs and other potentially injurious agents may have to be given, having been tested earlier, to patients in a more advanced stage of the illness. At this stage informed consent is not possible.

It has been suggested that all the ethical issues that might be foreseen could be discussed with tact and sensitivity, at the time of the diagnosis, with both the patient and his family when the patient, in a relatively insightful state, could address himself to the question of agreeing to, or rejecting, procedures that might be undertaken during the rest of the course of his illness. The idea of a 'penultimate will', in which the patient in the early stages of his illness designates members of his family or friends as legatees who will decide what might properly be done as he grows more seriously and helplessly ill, has also been considered. This would seem an attractive solution but the pressure being put on relatives might often become unacceptably great and the term executor might begin to assume a more sinister connotation for some people.

Whilst pondering upon these matters we would do well to remember that ultimately it is the views and values of society which will decide this issue as others have been determined in their time. We might do well to remember that when the ordinary public are confronted by the growing problem of dementia, changes might occur in attitudes – in the same way that the public decided that overpopulation and sexual freedom were incompatible with constraints on contraception and abortion – that will lead to a resolution of our difficulties without too much acrimony or fuss.

Huntington's chorea brings problems of a different kind to the ethical debate. The range of social and domestic difficulties associated with the illness have been detailed in earlier chapters and leave no doubt in anyone's mind that the condition is an extremely distressing one. There is no cure and no way of preventing the illness except by stopping the spread of the delinquent gene. The difficulties of doing this in diseased individuals are well appreciated. The impossible position the families of Huntington's choreics are placed in can be readily understood. Unlike with other causes of dementia, where the possibility of developing the same disease as the patient is relatively distant or non-existent, in Huntington's chorea there is a known and definite risk of affliction. At present there is little prospect of pre-natal diagnosis and the results of tests in asymptomatic carriers are equivocal. A foolproof test that might enable us to reassure non-carriers that they are safe is clearly a prospect devoutly to be wished. But what does one do with those one knows are doomed to disease and premature death, with much distress in between? If one believes those at risk would not wish to gamble with knowing their fates one will be very wrong. Reports from the USA (Stern and Eldridge, 1975), Britain (Barette and Marsden, 1979) and Australia (Teltcher and Polgar, 1981) have established that between 77% and 84% of respondents at risk, or with relatives with the disease, felt they would welcome a simple, safe and reliable test.

Fears have been expressed that those who would need to be told they could expect to have the disease might be devastated, go to pieces, squander their savings, abandon their plans, sink into depression and kill themselves. Perry (1981), a respected researcher into the condition, after detailing these dire consequences upon breaking the news to potential choreics, goes on to make this emphatic statement:

> I suggest that, pending development of an effective form of treatment, scientists who perform preclinical tests on persons at risk should ensure that the results of individual tests are not made available to those tested.

Earlier in his paper, Perry had quoted with approval Ingelfinger (1980), who had this to say in a more general context:

> A physician who merely spreads an array of vendibles in front of the patient and then says, 'go ahead and choose, it's your life', is guilty of shirking his duty, if not of malpractice. The physician . . . should list the alternatives and describe their pros and cons but then . . . [he] should recommend a specific course of action. He must take the responsibility, not shift it onto the shoulders of the patient.

The question of logic apart, these attitudes towards family members 'at risk' would suppose they were ignorant and somehow perversely irresponsible. Many members of the families of Huntington's choreics are as well informed as, if not better informed than, their professional advisers; they have day-to-day contact with patients and their knowledge of the condition is not academic but based on profound real-life experience, this life often being at best bothersome and at worst a variant of living hell. To deny potential carriers knowledge and then attempt to order their lives for them would, to many people, seem like patronizing, even insulting, conduct on the part of the doctor. Moreover, the days of authoritarian attitudes to patients and their families must surely have disappeared. And it would also seem highly improbable that those who agree, after some heart-searching, to undertake a test such as this would agree to go away empty-handed.

As with most matters in medical practice there can be no dogmatic laying down of rules. There is no great urgency in detecting a carrier state and the doctor can discuss the issue at some length with the subject, retailing the facts, outlining the pros and cons and offering reassurance where it can be given. The subject can then, if he does not want his fate revealed before time, withdraw *before* the test. If after this preparation the subject goes ahead with the test it will be more likely that he will be able to cope with a sombre outcome.

The problems of research into dementia are not confined to the search for suitable subject-matter or the efficient deployment of resources. Apart from the ethical issues associated with the investigation of the demented patient and the management of his condition, which are by themselves laudable aims and in keeping with traditions that have urged doctors to seek enlightenment and reduce suffering, we have to address ourselves to whether it is morally permissible to return treated demented patients into communities which may not be able, or willing, to provide for these patients. The growing number of dements, as we have seen in the historical survey, is a modern human problem. No other animal in this or any other age has so outlived its useful span of life and sunk into decrepitude in such numbers. In strictly biological terms it is unnecessary to live to the age when dementia becomes common. The basic natural requirements of a species to procreate and replace individuals is long met. The relatively more recent social requirement of productive labour ends between ages 60 and 65 and will in all probability be ended sooner that that in the near future. If human life ended by that age we would be faced with few dements and little need for any great concern. Our problems arise because individuals who have greatly exceeded both biological and social 'usefulness' go on living. If our research approaches to dementia bear fruit we shall be in a position to reverse these disease processes and return patients as fit individuals back into the community. Old patients will, however, return as old persons for there is no known method of making or keeping people young. Yet, what might be the kind of society that will receive these old persons? We have already considered the possibility of the elderly turning into a disadvantaged minority and must face the prospect that revolutionary advances in the medical management of dementia might well be a mixed blessing if we cannot assure that those sick individuals we proudly heal and return to society cannot be accepted by it. Absence of illness by itself does not guarantee a worthwhile human existence.

This is a more or less visionary preoccupation. A more practical exercise for the present is to worry about who should have the responsibility – financial, social and moral – for the demented. If the dementias are serious medical illnesses should the ultimate responsibility rest with the caring professions? Does the composition and outlook of the family in modern society place considerable and, perhaps, impossible strains on it when it is required to cope with patients with a serious and chronic illness of this kind? In the absence of a quite radical upheaval in the nature of family life in the future – which in turn might have serious social, financial and political repercussions – is it realistic to expect family care to be provided for growing numbers of demented patients?

And, yet, the alternative of state-underwritten, professionally provided care is not assured either. A popular phrase in situations like this is that 'political will' is required. We have already noted that there is moral basis to political action and the difficulties would seem daunting, but the greatest hope in a civilized democratic society must be that thinking and compassionate individuals within it can determine the intensity and direction of that will.

SUMMARY

(1) It is believed that about 10% of the population aged 65 and over are demented and half of them have severe dementia. Beyond age 80, 20% are affected and by age 85 a third of the population are thought to be demented. After this, the rates tend to level off.

(2) The prevalence of pre-senile dementia is probably a tenth of the numbers for senile dementia.

(3) On this basis there are over 715 000 senile dements now living in England and Wales. There will be a rise to about 760 000 cases in 1990 and there will be a slight fall after that.

(4) The change in age-structure (the relative numbers of persons over 80 years) is a more important factor than the absolute numbers in the population living beyond age 65.

(5) The incidence of dementia is less clear but varies from 0.5% per annum (case register studies) to 1.5% per annum (community surveys).

(6) Epidemiological research may well throw some light on aetiological factors.

(7) The prevalence of multi-infarct (vascular) dementia is around 10%. Huntington's chorea in general may range between 4 and 7 per 100 000 population. The incidence of idopathic normal pressure hydrocephalus is between 5% and 6% among pre-senile dements. Creutzfeldt–Jakob disease and Pick's disease are unusual and general paresis is now rare.

(8) For every demented patient being looked after in an institution (psychiatric and geriatric hospitals, local authority homes and private nursing homes) there are five living in the community. The provision of institutional day and inpatient places has fallen short of the officially recommended numbers.

(9)Demographic trends show that with a rise in the elderly population at risk, the problem of dementia will remain a serious one.

(10)Most dements belong to 'dependent' sections of the community and are at risk of becoming a disadvantaged minority facing prejudice.

(11)Social changes in modern society have altered the composition and attitudes of the family, and it is doubtful if the family can look after elderly dements without a great deal of stress and strain being imposed upon it.

(12)The financial cost to the community is a real one. The cost of keeping a demented patient in an institution is approaching £10 000 per year and the total cost of care for the demented elderly is already about £500 million annually. Care in the community is not always cheaper.

(13)It seems the most important factor affecting the patient's continued existence in the community is family support. Those who live by themselves are therefore at the greatest risk of being placed in an institution.

(14)The legal issues affecting elderly dements are those relating to criminal activity they might engage in, and those aspects of the law dealing with the protection of the patient and his property. The first, though of great interest, is of relatively little practical importance.

(15)The Mental Health Act and its amendments apply to the demented patient and the provisions for compulsory admission and care can be used in the normal way.

(16)Testamentary capacity assumes practical importance in the elderly dement and the Court of Protection enables the affairs of a patient to be looked after to his benefit.

(17)Some of the ethical issues considered are those relating to biopsy and invasive procedures on demented patients, the management of the pre-clinical state among carriers of the gene for Huntington's chorea and the wider question of whether it is moral to undertake research into sick old people who might not be welcome in society upon recovery or improvement in their condition. The attitudes of society, as manifested in a 'political will', are held to be important.

Further reading

(A full list of references is given at the end of the book)

Office of Health Economics (1979). *Dementia in Old Age*. (London)
Office of Health Economics (1980). *Huntington's Chorea*. (London)
Patrick, D.L. and Scrambler, G. (1982) (eds). *Sociology as Applied to Medicine*. (London: Bailliere Tindall)
Schoenberg, B.S. (1978), Neuroepidemiologic considerations in studies of Alzheimer's disease – senile dementia. In Katzman, R., Terry, R.D. and Bick, K.L. (eds). *Alzheimer's Disease: Senile Dementia and Related Disorders*. (New York: Raven Press)

11
A pathography of dementia

Babylon in all its desolation is a sight not so awful as that of the human mind in ruins

Scrope Davies (1783–1852)

A primary purpose of a pathography is to throw light on those areas of a distinguished person's life that might otherwise stay concealed from a casual reader's attention. This, as we shall soon see, was a not uncommon difficulty in the past. The truth is always relative but when the facts about the lives and works of the great came to be given out in a more discreet age than the present, there were as likely as not to be strenuous attempts made to keep knowledge of certain diseases away from public attention. Every age has decided the kind of morbidity that might be modish, and the biographer has taken it from there.

To the politician (and his family) especially, any whiff of syphilitic affection might have spelt ruin and an enduring stain on the family escutcheon. It is not difficult to understand therefore why the eminent historian A.L. Rowse, writing about Lord Randolph Churchill in *The Later Churchills* (1958), could not bring himself to discuss the dramatic fall from power and grace of Winston Churchill's father ('the most tragic career in British politics of the nineteenth century save Parnell's') in terms of any pathology. This was, of course, because the pathology being whispered abroad was cerebral syphilis. Instead, Rowse had to seek refuge in such aetiological factors as mercurial temperament, wayward genius and that staple of the English aristocracy, a weakness of moral fibre.

For its part, the *Encyclopaedia Britannica* considers seriously the opportunities (two, in its solemn judgement) that Nietzsche might have had to contract the syphilis which some years later would cripple his mind and body. And in 1922, the family of Lord Northcliffe went to great lengths to seek authoritative medical opinion which would refute the claims of numerous enemies that his terminal madness was due to syphilis.

185

Human nature being what it is, sensational details became a better aid to memory than more worthy but dull information about the subjects of biography. Very nearly everyone associates Henry VIII with multiple marriages and quarrels with the Pope, but relatively few would be able consciously to place an absolute ruler of England for nearly 40 years in a historical context even though he was a man whose wish, however distorted by his mental state, could well be a bloody and fateful command. And if a student of literature can learn about some aspects of general paresis from a life of Maupassant, this must be considered a painless method of health education.

Many of us are vicarious historians and few amongst us have not wondered what it must have been to live in times past. Every age has its preoccupations and obsessions and until well into this century – and even now in too many parts of the world – one of these was regarding sudden illness and early death. For several centuries until the present, syphilis was an occupational hazard for the bohemian artist as well as the more discreet but no less vulnerable statesman with the human touch. It is not unduly fanciful to suggest that if the Inland Revenue had existed in its present form, many of the lights of a bygone age, if they had deigned to pay taxes, could have demanded a rebate on the diverse variety of treatments they underwent for syphilis, often as much for a painless chancre as for a painful conscience.

The view that madness and creative genius go together as mutually sustaining phenomena is now held to be untenable. However, interest has persisted in trying to seek some elements which might be common to them both. Clearly, if the creative process is a product of the human mind, then intelligence and personality must have some bearing on the act of creation. By definition almost, creative works are abnormal and its creators are exceptional in not being normal, ordinary and mundane. We are not here interested, however, in the production of creative work which is the result of very high intelligence, exceptional creative ability or unusual traits of temperament but only in those which might be influenced by psychoses, of which the dementias are the organic representatives.

A case is made for manic depressive psychosis as being a condition potentially helpful to some artistic creation. In its depressive phase the illness leads to a marked retardation of psychic as well as other functions. The process of higher thought is slowed. Everything pauses, perhaps even halts. Then, like an awakening from hibernation, the patient recovers, often to normality, but occasionally progressing to the polar extreme of mania with its flight into psychic excess. There may well be a burst of stored creative energy. Perhaps the patient has not altogether been dormant in his depression, but creating subliminally, as in the synthetic phase of sleep, and out of reach of our inadequate methods of observation. The exuberance of excessive well-being probably helps him along.

Schizophrenia, on the other hand, is now believed to be destructive of the kind of creative work that is publicly appreciated and a full-blown schizophrenic cannot also be imagined in control of public affairs for very long in any society where a choice of leadership is available. Mad artists create in spite of, not because of, schizophrenia. Yet there might well be a

186

link between schizophrenia and the creative process though we have to dig beneath the surface for it. It appears a full complement of diseased genes predisposes to schizophrenia while a lesser number may give their owner the potential for exceptional creative ability. The sibs of floridly psychotic patients may thus be creative individuals. It seems artistic creation in some instances might be a controlled, constructive madness wrought by people who might be acceptably conventional in other avenues of life and able to fit into society without causing too much turmoil. So, Mr Anthony Burgess is invited to create a language for use in a feature film on life in pre-literate society; a patient using a language of his own manufacture would be deemed to show neologistic speech, a prime schizophrenic symptom.

Dementia, of course, is very different. A cardinal feature of the condition is loss of intellect and this must invariably curtail and then destroy creativity. Productive artists and active public figures who have become demented have been cut off in their prime. Most dementias, however, affect the elderly and in many instances their creative lives are past. They have usually retired from public and professional life and their decline, whilst painfully apparent to those close to them, rarely becomes known to the public until, usually, a sensational biography makes an impact. The exceptions were Messrs Gladstone and Winston Churchill, both in office on or after their 80th year, with the latter showing signs of physical and mental disability. But a tenth of dementias occur in those not aged 65 and it will be mainly this group who will form the subjects for discussion in this chapter.

Preoccupation with the mental stability of leaders of great states has once again become fashionable. There were no universally deadly weapons to tempt unstable rulers in Tudor England but the powers of the King then were absolute. Ove Brinch (1974) has considered the life of Henry VIII (1491–1548) with special reference to the mental changes that came about in his middle age. Henry, son of Henry VII, the first of the Tudor Kings, was born in 1491 and mounted the throne in April 1509 when his father died. The 18-year-old Henry VIII was 6 feet tall, possessed a fine physique and a 'pleasing countenance', well-educated, well-read, fluent in several languages, an accomplished composer and performer on several musical instruments, a keen hunter and sportsman, charming, friendly and the richest King in Christendom. At the age of 23 he developed a skin lesion which was feared might be smallpox but it lasted 2 months and faded away without leaving pock-marks. Brinch believes it might have been a syphilitic lesion. This was, of course, the time soon after Columbus had returned from the New World with the syphilitic spirochaete and the infection had begun to ravage all Europe. The infection was no respecter of persons and it is clear, even without the elaborate attempts that are usually made to trace the 'source', the King and his court would have been highly susceptible.

The King is said to have started to suffer from severe, recurrent headaches from the age of 37. The next significant incident in his medical history seems to have taken place in his 44th year when an ulcer appeared on one of his legs. This seems never to have healed and every so often turned into a painful fistula. It is now believed that this ulcer might have begun life as a syphilitic gumma. About the same age he seems to have acquired a

187

deformity of the right side of his nose with a deviation of the nasal septum, again a possible syphilitic complication.

In his fifties Henry was virtually incapable of walking, partly because of his gross obesity but chiefly, it is thought, owing to weakness of his legs and evidence for this is adduced from several portraits of the time which show him standing on a wide base.

While these physical features were setting in, from about his 40th year the charming, intellectual, sociable and well-balanced youth was turning into the cruel, egotistical and tyrannical megalomaniac of his last 17 years. A reign of terror and execution was unleashed in the kingdom and various quarrels with Rome became a major obsession. He had started to suffer from paroxysmal fits of rage and was amnesic for these episodes. His memory, especially for recent events, began to suffer and on one occasion it was noted with consternation that he had given written orders to tear down the French forts around Boulogne while issuing simultaneous verbal orders to leave them untouched.

While the memory and changes and personality disorganization seem to be conclusive there seems to have been little evidence of gross intellectual change till the very last weeks. However, orders were given, and followed, for executions. Henry ordered the execution of the Earl of Surrey and his father, Norfolk, for allegedly plotting against him. Surrey was beheaded 8 days before the decrepit King finally died but Norfolk was saved by Henry's death the evening before his execution.

Brinch's conclusion, with the inevitable rider that we are considering scanty evidence at second hand after four centuries, is that Henry had neurosyphilis, possibly taboparetic in nature. A complication in this case was that the King drank excessively, too, and some of the mental changes, especially those with regard to memory disturbance, might have had an alcoholic basis as well.

The crucial issue that must arise in any pathographic consideration of Henry VIII is what might happen when a ruler with absolute power underwent the serious and, for practical purposes, irreversible changes of dementia and yet no person or institution could modify or correct his excesses. Winston Churchill (1874–1965) lived in a vastly different age and could not, even if he had so desired, aspire to absolute power, but more than any man in Britain in modern times he came near to indispensability as the war-time Prime Minister.

Popular belief has it that Churchill showed his greatest disability during his peace-time premiership between 1951 and 1955 and thereafter. This is undeniably true but as Lord Moran (1966), Churchill's personal physician, and L'Etang (1970) have confirmed, the signs were there before, beginning in the later years of the war. Moran has said it was Churchill's exhaustion of mind and body that accounts for much that is inexplicable in his conduct of the last year of the war, including the deterioration in his relations with Roosevelt. L'Etang quotes Alanbrooke, the Chief of the Imperial General Staff, as having noted in March 1944 that Churchill was incapable of concentrating for even a few minutes and his mind kept wandering. He attributed this state to the effects of recurrent attacks of pneumonia

Churchill had suffered just previously. In May 1944 the Polish Ambassador recorded Churchill's difficulty in grasping what was being told him, and he and several other observers at that time wondered if 'over-tiredness' could be the cause.

While with hindsight we might reasonably suppose these were prodromal symptoms, there was still no unequivocal evidence of cerebrovascular disease. In 1947 Lord Moran, whilst noting the vaguer manifestations of normal senility, could also record that the now 73-year-old Leader of the Opposition showed retinal arteriopathy: 'There is plenty of evidence that his circulation was sluggish', says Moran, but does not provide any futher evidence.

The first dramatic event occurred in August 1949 in Monte Carlo, when after a night at cards Churchill complained of weakness in his right hand. Sensation was affected, as was gait. It was a mild stroke with little residual deficit and the docile public in that innocent age was easily kept in the dark. A year later Churchill had an episode of 'sudden mistiness' and a couple of years after that there was an episode of transient speech difficulty. Thus, when he returned as Prime Minister in 1951, there was much clearer evidence of cerebrovascular disease. Moran had no doubt the 77-year-old Prime Minster was greatly changed. The enormous capacity for work which he had shown in the past seemed to have gone – indeed the PM's office reported that he was not doing his work – as had his self-confidence. Everything had become an effort and he was forgetting his figures. The Prime Minister's private secretary noted that five-page documents had to be reduced to a paragraph for Churchill and the Queen's private secretary confirmed, L'Etang observes, that Churchill could not follow the trend of a discussion.

Churchill, however, resisted all moves to persuade him to step down and the chosen heir, Anthony Eden, had a frustrating wait until 1955. One of the chief difficulties in the way of appreciating the seriousness of the situation was that the patient denied it was serious or refused to talk about it, and no-one would or could bell this particularly intractable cat!

The major cerebrovascular episode during Churchill's term of office occurred in June 1953 at a dinner for the visiting Italian Prime Minister. Churchill had developed a right-sided weakness, inarticulate speech, an unsteady gait which portrayed drunkenness to the distinguished guests. Two days later the weakness spread to the left arm. Things looked grave and his doctors wondered if he would survive the year. Yet his mental faculties at the time were still largely intact and Moran thought his patient replied to the Queen's best wishes, 5 days after the stroke, 'with . . . poise, proportion and [a] sense of detachment'. The underlying seriousness of the situation could not be denied, however, and Moran thought Churchill was 'really living on a volcano' and not one of his medical attendants seemed to have any doubt he was unfit to continue as Prime Minister.

But he defied them all and within a couple of months was chairing a Cabinet meeting. Within a further few months he had impressively addressed the Conservative Party Conference, answered questions in the House of Commons and attended a summit meeting in Bermuda. But the recovery was apparent, not real, and L'Etang reports that Churchill no longer studied state papers but read novels and played interminable games of bezique.

The mental changes were to be seen more prominently after this time. By the summer of the next year it was said Churchill could no longer follow discussion in Cabinet and in the autumn of 1954, in contrast to his performance of the previous year, he made a disastrous speech to the Tory conference. At the end of that year, following some extraordinary but unsustainable claims he had made regarding the conduct of the last phases of the war which embarrassed the Government, he had to apologize to the House of Commons. It was clear he was tripping over words and names of people, confusing Eisenhower with Adenauer on one occasion. He was finally persuaded to step down in 1955 but stayed in the Commons till 1964 and died a year later, much of time since giving up the leadership being spent in silence and immobility.

The criticism has been made, especially of Lord Moran, that many of these observations were noted when Churchill, as a result of a bout of illness, was at his worst. Indeed, more recent evidence, including Cabinet papers recently made public, seems to suggest that Churchill, though certainly never in anything approaching even reasonable health, was not at all times incapable of running public affairs. These views of him are not incompatible, and may be equally valid, for Churchill appears to have had a condition which runs a notoriously episodic course. That this illness was of arteriosclerotic or vascular origin there seems little doubt. But whether a diagnosis of dementia can be upheld for Churchill's condition prior to 1955 is uncertain, though it is clear that the disability in his last years amounted to dementia. The motor weakness and the speech deficit were in all probability focal lesions and the malaise, lack of interest and physical weakness, all features of his tenure of 10 Downing Street, could be attributed to the effects of a serious illness. It is interesting that in between major episodic attacks Churchill was able to function at some level, the disability after each attack persisting roughly at the same level until the next episode intervened, the so-called 'step-wise' progression of the disease.

It was 20 years before the advent of computerized tomography and there was no autopsy, so the lesions could not be visualized. The diagnosis must rest on the evidence of the reports of significant higher dysfunction as a result of presumed cerebrovascular disease.

Churchill's father, Lord Randolph Churchill, had a meteoric rise to fame and power and then an equally spectacular fall. Lord Randolph (1849–1895) died when Winston was 21. Father and son seem to have shared an uneasy relationship and were never close. Lord Randolph entered the Commons in 1874, a few months before Winston was born, and soon made his mark with a series of brilliant and scathing speeches, a particular target being old Mr Gladstone. The first signs of serious ill health seem to have surfaced in 1882 when he missed 5 months in the Commons because of an illness, very likely depression. The Churchills, father and son, were prone to depressive spells, made famous by Winston's accounts of his 'Black Dog'. In the summer of 1885, having made a recovery of sorts, Lord Randolph found himself as Secretary for India in Lord Salisbury's government. Queen Victoria apparently had some misgivings about this appointment. The government soon fell in 1886 but Salisbury returned to form his second administration later that year and to the consternation of the Queen suggested Lord Randolph might be given even more responsible office. Anita Leslie records the Queen's observations: '. . . .[Lord Salisbury] feared Lord Randolph Churchill must be Chancellor of the Exchequer and Leader [of the House of Commons] which I did not like. He is so mad and odd and has also bad health . . . '

His recovery from illness was still not complete and he was apt to be nervous and lacked confidence. A sparkling speaker, he now found speech-making difficult but could yet rise to the occasion. He was, however, only 37 years old, the youngest man to hold such senior office since the younger Pitt, and there seemed no limit to what he might rise to.

Just before Christmas of that year, however, on some relatively trivial matter concerning defence expenditure, he resigned. It was not so much his going but the manner of it that outraged virtually everyone. He had sent his resignation letter to Lord Salisbury with a copy to *The Times*. A distinctly unamused Queen Victoria learned of her minister's resignation, as did her subjects, in the next morning's newspaper. Unaccountably, Lord Randolph had self-destructed.

There was little prospect of his ever making a comeback even if he had regained the best of health. But as Anita Leslie notes, there was a steady decline from now on. He seemed tense, irritable and unpredictable; his financial judgement faltered and his extravagance led to mounting debts. Over the next few years a multiplicity of symptoms – palpitations, dizziness, vertigo, deafness and unsteady fingers – affected him and his speeches in the House were but shades of those glorious ones in the past. He looked terribly haggard and his words were often inaudible and incoherent. His hand-writing had become unsteady too.

He spoke in the House for the last time in June 1894. It was an appalling speech in which he lost the thread of the argument and had to be prompted by fellow members. Soon afterwards he left on a world cruise, haggard, semi-articulate and by now showing an extremely labile mood. He was being given 6 months to live. Leslie quotes from a letter written by his devoted wife, Jennie:

> Physically he is better but mentally he is 1000 times worse. Even his mother wishes now that he had died the other day . . . up to now the General Public and even society does not know the real truth . . . it would do incalculable harm to his political reputation.

Mercifully, the end came quietly on 24 January 1895.

Quite clearly, a malignant pathological process, different in chronicity and intensity than in his son 60 years later, was at work. Interestingly, the disease seems to have set in with nervous features – depression, anxiety or a mixture of the two – that he had tended to show even before his terminal illness but this time he never regained good health. The quite insightless

191

political behaviour – it seems he never appreciated the nature of his actions or his insult to the Queen – took place in the midst, it would appear, of his last sickness and it was not very long before anyone who was close to Lord Randolph could see he was mortally ill.

A half-century after Lord Randolph's fall, and as his son was preparing to depart into the political wilderness, another British Prime Minister was showing signs of dementia in office. James Ramsay MacDonald (1866–1937) was Britain's first Labour Prime Minister, for 9 months in 1924, and then head of the National Government between 1929 and 1935. In 1927, aged 61 and on a visit to the USA, he developed a mysterious throat infection which kept him in hospital for a month and off work for 5 months. David Marquand (1977) in his definitive biography describes how Ramsay Macdonald's signs of ageing could be traced to this episode. Five years later glaucoma affected first one eye and then the other, and ageing and fatigue worsened. He had returned completely exhausted from a disarmament conference in Geneva and had noted:

'My trouble . . . is just a complete breakdown from top to toe, inside and out. . . .' A visitor found him 'rather woolly' and noted a rapid weakening of his physical and mental powers from about this time. Always prone to insomnia and bouts of unhappiness, he was now subject to spells amounting to depression. Marquand describes how in early 1933 Ramsay MacDonald was seen looking nervously over his shoulder in the middle of a speech in the House of Commons. Later he explained that he had thought that a man in the gallery was about to shoot at him. In Geneva, around the same time, he had lost consciousness briefly while making a speech and did not know what he was saying.

His speech soon became confused. Once, replying to an intervention in the House, he had said:

> He thinks that he is the only impatient man in this House to get things done. I will beat him 50 per cent any day he likes. . . No doubt he has a hawk-like desire for action, without bridle and without saddle, across the Atlantic.

The difficulties with his speech were quite apparent to him and Marquand records how Ramsay MacDonald would lie awake at nights before speeches and then torture himself with their memory afterwards. He made notes in his diary:

> Cannot be done. Like man flying in mist: can fly all right but cannot see the course. . . .

> Machine run down: stupid mind and can do no work and sick in body. . . .

> . . . very tired and stupid . . . head a mere log, no memory, no energy, yawning all day.

The public, ever eager to attribute mental failings to scandalous causes, were being urged to consider the idea that the Prime Minister's mental and physical decline might be due to the strain of being blackmailed by a prostitute in Central Europe. Marquand considers this to have been unlikely. Whatever Ramsay MacDonald or the prostitute might have picked up, he continued to decline and by October–November 1934 his performance in Cabinet had begun to deteriorate as well. In 1935 he resigned as Prime Minister but continued as Lord President of the Council in Baldwin's Cabinet, 'a forlorn, lost and helpless figure, eliciting no sympathy', forever doomed as a 'traitor' to the Labour Movement. Even his golf and handwriting deteriorated, and his diary entries often became marred by spelling mistakes and omitted words. In conversation he made slips of the tongue and forgot people's names. He resigned with the Baldwin Cabinet in 1937 and died at sea later that year.

Ramsay MacDonald's deterioration took place over 6 years and, as with Lord Randolph Churchill, began with depressive and nervous symptoms but there seems little doubt that the illness then ran a predominantly organic course. The type of speech disturbance is good evidence for that, and it is interesting that expressive speech disorder of the kind Ramsay MacDonald exhibited is associated with a particularly poor prognosis in certain kinds of senile dementia.

Thus, three controversial political figures, spanning three political generations, have contrived to show, as far as we are able to say from published work, three major forms of dementing illness. What influence their illness had on their political judgement must always remain a matter for conjecture. Winston Churchill, at one time in the 1930s the most reviled politician in Britain, rose to a position of reverence 5 momentous years later, and had established his reputation before he became seriously unwell; his faulty judgement lay in postponing his departure. Lord Randolph's outrageous behaviour and his gratuitous insult to Queen Victoria and his colleagues, when he was perhaps but a step away from the Tory leadership, doomed him; it is not unlikely he was harbouring the early stages of general paresis within him at the time. And as for Ramsay MacDonald, the alleged traitor of the working class, it is again likely that the disease process, which we may surmise was senile dementia of the Alzheimer type, had already taken over his brain as he formed his second administration. Would the course of history have been very different if these men did not have their incapacity?

William Somerset Maugham (1874–1965), the most widely read novelist since Dickens, was an almost exact contemporary of Winston Churchill's, even to the extent of being able to remark when it was suggested he might be *non compos*, 'If you think I am ga-ga, you should look at Winston'.

Despite his great fame, wealth and superficial charm, Maugham was a deeply troubled man, harbouring feelings of being unloved and being unable to love, futility, envy (of those who were happy) and possessed of a façade of normality that masked homosexual guilt. But he survived old age well, sustained physically by the rejuvenating injections of Paul Niehans. It was not until his 87th year that mental decline could be detected.

We now have Ted Morgan's (1980) definitive biography of Maugham and the first sign was thought to have been Maugham's obsession with the safety of his valuable collection of paintings at his Villa Mauresque following the theft of a Goya from the National Gallery in London. Shortly after this, in the presence of his daughter and grandchildren, he began muttering, shouting and cursing. These attacks were episodic, and in between them he was thought to be normal. It transpired that Maugham had been having attacks of this kind for over a year, when he would rave about imaginary enemies, shout and scream, and throw water and furniture about. Often he required sedation.

The pictures had become a bone of contention between father and daughter. A sale at Sotheby's was followed by the firm being sued by the daughter for her share of the proceeds. His decline continued, he shouted obscenities at visitors and confused some old friends with his daughter.

Then came an episode that cost Maugham a good deal of public sympathy. Persuaded by the *Sunday Express*, he wrote a serial on his life. It included a tasteless, even scurrilous, attack on his dead wife Syrie and created a storm that made him even more distant from his daughter. Noel Coward, an old and close friend, was led to remark 'The man who wrote that awful slop is not the man who has been my friend . . . .some evil spirit has entered his body. He is dangerous, a creature to be feared and shunned' (quoted by Morgan, 1980).

That same year (1962) he became convinced that his daughter was going to have him certified as incompetent to manage his affairs, and in order to forestall this he adopted Alan Searle, his secretary, companion and lover. His daughter challenged this decision and won the case. The effect on Maugham seemed to be an acceleration in his decline. His behaviour continued to be bizarre. As some distinguished visitors came to see him they found Maugham emerging from behind the sofa adjusting his trousers, having defaecated on the rug, and scooping up a handful of faeces. One night he left his home without his shoes and wondered down a dangerously busy road. His hearing and his sight faded fast and he could read no longer. He woke up screaming in the middle of the night. When his daughter came to visit him – the Sotheby case being settled out of court – he could not recognize her and thought she was his much reviled, dead wife. The amazing thing, though, was his physical prowess. The body, topped up by rejuvenating fluids, showed no signs of decline.

On some days he was still lucid and could even give reasonable interviews, talking about the past even though recent years were a blank. Early in 1965 he contracted double pneumonia but his remarkably fit body helped him recover. Then in December of that year he fell three times in quick succession, slipped into a coma and died in hospital, though his body was spirited away to avoid autopsy and his death was reported from home.

Maugham declined from that time of life when over a third of the population would expect to dement. His symptoms were distressing and were to be seen in the devastating decline in higher (and in Maugham they were high) functions and in the cruel caricature of his never very agreeable personality. The physical body stood the course, almost unscathed, till the very end. In this – perhaps it was really due to rejuvenation – Maugham differed from most senile dements.

Somerset Maugham learned his short story-telling craft from the man who made the modern commercial story, Guy de Maupassant (1850–1893), who was destined to die before he was 43 years old. Maupassant's mother, who might have been Flaubert's mistress, was always a nervous and depressed woman who had an exophthalmic goitre, which Maupassant might later have had himself. Unlike many of the great whose syphilitic infections have to be presumed, Maupassant himself is able to throw light on the primary infection. At the age of 27, in some triumph, he writes 'I have caught the real pox, the pox that Francis I died from'.

Two comprehensive accounts of Maupassant's decline, by Ignotus (1966) and Lerner (1975), are available. They show that around the age of 33 Maupassant's eyes had become so weak he could hardly read or write, and was forced into pressing his friends to do his proof-reading for him. An eye specialist believed his eye condition was related to the syphilitic infection. A year or so later, his valet reported, he was having occasional hallucinatory experiences of a double of his sitting in a chair or being reflected in a mirror. It is interesting that several of Maupassant's short stories written at the time seem to have references to abnormal experiences including hallucinations, and also contain premonitions of impending death.

In 1887, when Maupassant was 37 years old, his brother Herve, who seems to have been retarded, fell ill, and by the following year started to show signs of the madness that culminated in his death at the age of 33. He is now also thought to have had general paresis. In that same year Maupassant developed pains in his abdomen, suffered from crippling headaches and was ordered to rest. Already he had grandiose and persecutory ideas. He looked thin and haggard and the writer de Goncourt recorded in his diary 'he is not destined, it would seem, to live to a great age'.

Maupassant became depressed, was hardly ever out of pain and had temporary spells of blindness. Several diagnoses, including syphilis, were being mentioned. He had become very irritable and bad-tempered, suspicious and sensitive, but continued to work. Memory difficulties were first noted in 1890 when he began to stammer as well. Excerpts from his letters, quoted by Lerner, reflect his torment.

> I have just spent the night getting up and going to bed again haunted by nightmares, visions and imaginary noises. . . .

> I am virtually blind . . . .very depressed.

> I think it is the beginning of my death agony. I have almost lost the use of speech. . . .

On one occasion, as he walked near a cemetery, he was convinced he had come face to face with a ghost of himself.

Lerner quotes from a letter Maupassant wrote to a doctor in 1891:

> I am utterly without hope. I am in my death agony. I have a softening of the brain brought on by my bathing my notrils with salt-water. The salt has fermented in my brain and every night my brains are dripping through my nose and mouth in a sticky paste. . . . It means Death is

near and I am going mad. My head is all confused. Goodbye, dear friend, you will not be seeing me again....

He decided to shoot himself to kill the flies devouring the salt in his brain. His valet, who had seen him fire through the window at an imaginary enemy, secretly took out the bullets. Thwarted, that very night Maupassant cut his throat, calling out theatrically 'Look what I have done. . . . I have cut my throat . . . there is no doubt I am going insane.' He was unsuccessful and soon went berserk and was taken to a private clinic in a straitjacket.

Until the last 6 months he alternated between periods of confused thought and irrational behaviour and shorter spells of normality when he would read the newspapers and stroll in the clinic's grounds.

As the year passed it was reported that 'Maupassant begins to turn into an animal', being presumably a reference to his howling and licking the walls of his room. At other times he was accusing people of embezzling his money and plagiarizing his work. He was convinced he was God's son by his mother, refused to part with his urine, claiming it contained diamonds, and was obsessed by the idea of piles of eggs and constantly mentioned his train journey to Purgatory and his dialogue with Lucifer about taking over the world.

By Easter of 1893 he was suffering from fits, during one of which he hurled a billiard ball at another inmate. Within a couple of months he had sunk into a coma following violent convulsions and died in July 1893, just before his 43rd birthday.

Maupassant, the creative artist, seems to have had florid psychopathology, and the question needs to be asked if the content of the symptoms of dementia depend of the richness of the imagination that is perverted and later destroyed by the disease. It seems likely that some of the stories Maupassant wrote in the early or prodromal phases of his illness had a basis in what he was experiencing at the time, and some critics have observed a growing preoccupation in his works about 'another self' and also forebodings of death.

A creative artist in another mode whose symptomatology seemed influenced by his creativity – a form of occupational dementia, it might be suggested – was Robert Schumann (1810–1856), on whose medical history light was thrown by Eliot Slater (1976). It was not always held that Schumann became demented through general paresis. In fact, until the middle of this century the view was that he had a functional psychosis, schizophrenia or manic-depressive illness, on which an organic process somehow supervened in the last 2 years. Tracing the medical chronology of Schumann's life, Slater believes now that all the nervous symptoms which troubled Schumann from the ages of about 18 to 42 were manic-depressive. These seem to include several episodes of depressive illness, some of several months' duration, and a few bouts in which elation appears to have been the predominant state. Schumann survived them all without any deterioration of personality, which argues against the schizophrenic hypothesis.

The premonitory symptoms of organic brain disease may have been noted in 1843 and 1844, when he had giddiness and tinnitus, though Schumann never had Menière's disease. In 1850 and 1852 there were pains in his feet, and in the latter year burning sensations at the back of his head and a succession of prickling nervous sensations in the backbone and fingertips were reported. Also in 1852, when he was 42, difficulties with speech and a fit were observed, and Schumann had to give up conducting. A year later a congestive attack was noted and speech and auditory symptoms were becoming more prominent. In February 1854 Schumann had reported a painful ear which progressed to tinnitus. Four days later he put down a paper saying he could not read any more as he kept hearing the note A. Within a week the musical tones had developed into angelic music, 'magnificent music, with instruments of spendid resonance, the like of which has never been heard on earth before'. The morning after the angel voices were transformed into the voices of devils who told him he was a sinner and would be thrown into hell. A continuous state of auditory and visual hallucination continued for weeks but his consciousness was preserved at least partly, and he could recognize and speak to his wife. Soon he was overcome by intense feelings of guilt and remorse, kept repeating he would go to hell and must never stop reading the Bible, all of which suggest a depressive condition. He wanted to be taken to the lunatic asylum, left his house inadequately clothed against a storm and was brought back after being fished out of the Rhine. He was now taken to an asylum. His delirium seems to have resolved and he settled, though very soon agitation took over. Within a couple of months there was another psychotic phase with hallucinations accusing him of plagiarism and confused speech. He refused to eat, presumably because he thought he might be poisoned, but then recovered. He continued to be changeable with periods of clarity and confusion alternating. He continued to scribble illegibly, his recent memory was almost non-existent and on one occasion he threw some wine he was drinking to the floor, saying it was poisoned. The musical hallucinations continued, his speech and writing became incoherent, he deteriorated very rapidly and died on 29 July 1856 after a day of continuous convulsion.

The almost irrelevant detail of how and when the primary syphilitic lesion was acquired seems to be available for Schumann. An injury to a finger in his early twenties, which affected his piano playing, might have been due, it is now thought, to the mercurial treatment of a syphilitic lesion.

Schumann's autopsy findings became available in 1873. Amongst other findings there was considerable atrophy of the brain and general paresis was suggested for the first time, but when attempts were made to check the hospital records they had mysteriously disappeared. It took nearly another hundred years before Eliot Slater and Alfred Meyer could say in 1959 that 'on careful consideration [no alternative diagnosis] could fit all the facts as well as syphilitic disease . . . a combination of cerebrospinal syphilis and dementia paralytica'.

While Schumann incubated his fatal illness, Friedrich Wilhelm Nietzsche (1844–1900) was being born in Saxony in 1844 into a family with strong religious connections. Nietzsche's father died when Nietzsche was 5. There is some suspicion that it might have been following general paresis. Nietzsche's health was always indifferent – headaches, pain in the eyes, hoarseness, rheumatism, insomnia, led him to write: 'my health from day to day is pitiable' – and he would have made a classic subject for a study on 'creative malady'. Much of his early writing is about the state of his health and he was a frequenter of spas for health cures; in 1876 he took a whole year off as sick leave. In 1879 he resigned his chair in classical philology at Basle because of his health and became increasingly solitary. '. . . I am a headache-plagued half-lunatic, crazed by too much solitude'.

He was suicidal but carried on, and the first whiff of fame seemed to come his way. In Turin in 1888, where earlier he had one of his rare periods of relative peace and contentment, a visitor noted, 'Nietzsche seemed to drag himself along with difficulty . . . and his speech often became slurred, heavy and halting'. Another writer felt a letter written in October that year showed the 'first unmistakeable signs of madness'. He fell in the streets of Turin one day, and the process of breakdown accelerated from then on. Early in 1889 he created a scene in a square in Turin by embracing a horse, and was brought back to Basle. He ceased talking that day and his memory was lost too. He seemed to enjoy music and understood what was read to him, and could utter sudden cries of pain, which might have meant a response to 'lightning pains'. He sat, gentle and childlike, in a 'continuous reverie', nursed for 12 years first by his mother and then his sister. The firm diagnosis of dementia paralytica was made at the time. Nietzsche, acclaimed later as Germany's most influential philosopher, died on 25 August 1900.

If Maupassant and Schumann had allowed their art to creep into their symptoms, Nietzsche, the tormented introvert, suffered in silence.

References and further reading

HENRY VIII
Brinch, O. (1974). The medical problems of Henry VIII. In Sorsby, A. (ed.)   *Tenements of Clay*. (London: Julian Friedmann)

WINSTON CHURCHILL
L'Etang, H. (1970). *The Pathology of Leadership*. (London: William   Heinemann)
Moran, Lord (1966). *Winston Churchill. The Struggle for Survival 1940-   1965*. (London: Constable)

LORD RANDOLPH CHURCHILL
Leslie, A. (1969). *Jennie. The Life of Lady Randolph Churchill*. (London: Hutchinson)

J. RAMSAY MACDONALD
Marquand, D. (1977). *Ramsay MacDonald*. (London: Jonathan Cape)

W. SOMERSET MAUGHAM
Morgan, T. (1980). *Somerset Maugham*. (London: Jonathan Cape)

GUY DE MAUPASSANT
Ignotus, P. (1966). *The Paradox of Maupassant*. (London: University of   London Press)
Lerner, M.G. (1975). *Maupassant*. (London: George Allen and Unwin)

ROBERT SCHUMANN
Slater, E. (1976). Schumann's illness. In Walker, A. (ed.). *Robert Schumann: The Man and his Music*. (London: Faber and Faber)

Appendix: The clinical assessment of the patient suspected of being demented

The purpose of the clinical assessment of a patient is fourfold.

(1) To determine whether or not he is demented.
(2) To seek a cause for the dementia.
(3) To be able to give a prognosis.
(4) To be in a position to plan future management.

Step 2 usually requires psychometric assessment and investigations in addition to clinical assessment.

THE HISTORY

This is taken in the usual way, and the importance of an account by a reliable independent informant is emphasized.

After the onset, duration and evolution of each symptom has been noted, it is necessary to question the informant as to the extent to which symptoms have affected the patient's day-to-day behaviour. The headings used in the Crichton Geriatric Behavioural Rating Scale, such as mobility, orientation, communication, co-operation, restlessness, dressing, feeding, continence and sleep may be used to assess the changes in the patient's behaviour and, if possible, a rough quantitative assessment can be made.

The family history would pay special attention to mental and nervous illness in the family, especially of a hereditary nature, which might have led to incarceration and death in institutions, or suicide.

Personal history must include an account of education, occupational level and retirement. An assessment of the intellectual level at which the patient functioned can be made at this time. Some assessment of an existing marriage and the quality of the relationship with the spouse, children and sibs is necessary.

Previous medical history must take note of a past history of psychiatric

199

illness. A history of past depressive illness or alcoholism may be significant. The intake of drugs, prescribed and unprescribed, needs to be noted.

Premorbid personality assessment is even more important than the assessment of intellectual functioning in health at this stage in the history, as no further information is likely to be obtained. The fact that the examiner seeks to know something about the personality *before* it underwent change must be emphasized to relatives and friends. How has the patient changed? What was he like previously? The areas of personality functioning that may be considered are ability to look after himself, interests (both intellectual and practical), energy and drive, concern for others, equable mood and good temper, relating to people and the extent to which he could trust others. The nature and extent of any change is noted separately.

PHYSICAL EXAMINATION

This is carried out in the usual way, and though the nervous system is obviously important, as every system can contribute to the changes of dementia, a full examination is necessary. Allowance must be made for the changes of age on physical signs, and the examiner must beware of false-positive and false-negative signs (see Chapter 2).

MENTAL AND COGNITIVE STATE EXAMINATION

The mental state examination of appearance and general behaviour, mood, abnormal beliefs and abnormal experiences is carried out in the usual way.

A more comprehensive examination of speech function than is under taken usually is necessary. Note the presence of dysarthria and aphasia. In the latter case spoken and written speech, in terms of both comprehension and production, need to be assessed.

The assessment of cognitive function begins with attention and concen tration. The extent to which they are affected needs to be noted and a more objective test is 'serial sevens' forwards and backwards. Orientation is dealt with next, and after that memory. Some idea of the patient's memory and intellectual function may have been obtained during history-taking. Immediate and short-term memory may be assessed by giving the patient a name and address and getting him to repeat it immediately and 5 minutes later. To test non-verbal memory a simple geometric figure is shown the patient, and he is asked to reproduce it immediately and 5 minutes afterwards.

The clinical assessment of intelligence, a notoriously unreliable business, is probably best done with regard to the pre-morbid history of the patient and by taking account of his educational achievements, his occupational level and previous general interests. The interpretation of proverbs is thought to be a guide to abstract reasoning, and can be tried.

An assessment must also be made of other cortical dysfunctions. Visuospatial function is tested by getting the patient to copy a series of simple geometric figures directly and from memory. Visual agnosia and prosopagnosia (defective recognition of faces) is then tested, as is apraxia, topographical disorientation, right–left disorientation and finger agnosia.

If indicated on this clinical assessment, a referral to a psychologist follows. Armed with the psychometric report the clinician can approach the following questions. (He could try the questions immediately after the clinical assessment but his answers might be slightly less securely based.)

1. Is the patient demented?

Is his condition acquired with the presence of global deficits in clear consciousness? Is there a decline in intellectual level and memory functioning leading to behavioural disturbance and social disorganization?

If so, in terms of the discussion in Chapter 2, the patient is demented.

2. How severe is the dementia and is it progressing?

A clinical assessment on examination and follow-up will enable this question to be answered. A slightly more formal arrangement, which takes in most of the questions asked during the clinical interview, is discussed by Hodkinson (1973) and is shown in the table. A cut-off point of 25 is said to distinguish between normals and dements. An idea of severity can be obtained by its use on follow-up. Alternatively, repeat psychometry may indicate progression of the dementia.

The Mental Test Score (from Hodkinson, 1973)

	Score
Name	0/1
Age	0/1
Time (to nearest hour)	0/1
Time of day	0/1
Name and address for 5 min. recall	0/5 (2 – name, 2 – street, 1 – town)
Day of week	0/1
Date (correct day of month)	0/1
Month	0/1
Year	0/1
Place: Type of place	0/1
Name of Hospital	0/1
Ward	0/1
Town	0/1
Recognition of two persons	0/1
Date of birth (day and month)	0/1
Place of birth (town)	0/1
School attended	0/1
Former occupation	0/1
Name of wife, sib, or next of kin	0/1
Date of World War I (years)	0/1
Date of World War II (years)	0/1
Name of present Monarch	0/1
Name of present Prime Minister	0/1
Months of year backwards	0/2
Count 1–20	0/2
Count 20–1	0/2

34 (maximum)

3. Can a cause of the dementia be found?

Here the results of various investigations will supplement the clinical findings noted in Chapter 3.

4. Has all the information been assembled to draw up a formulation?

The discussion in Chapter 2 is a guide to this.

References

Adams, R.D., Fisher, C.M., Hakim, S., Ojemann, R. and Sweet, W. (1965). Symptomatic occult hydrocephalus with "normal" cerebrospinal fluid: a treatable syndrome. *N. Engl. J. Med.*, **273**, 117-126

Albert, M.L. (1978). Subcortical dementia. In Katzman, R., Terry, R.D. and Bick, K.L. (eds). *Alzheimer's Disease: Senile Dementia and Related Disorders*. (New York: Raven Press)

Albert, M.S. (1981). Geriatric neuropsychology. *J. Consult. Clin. Psychol.*, **49** (6), 835-850

Alexander, D.A. (1972). Senile dementia: a changing perspective. *Br. J. Psychiatry*, **121**, 207-214

Alzheimer, A. (1907). Ueber eine eigenartige Erkrankung der Hirnrinde. *Allg. Z. Psychiatrie*, **64**, 146-148 (Tr. R.H. Wilkins and I.A. Brody (1969). *Arch. Neurol.*, **21**, 109-110)

American Psychiatric Association (1978). *Diagnostic and Statistical Manual of Mental Disorders*. III. (Washington, DC: American Psychiatric Association)

Anderson, E.W. and Mallison, W.P. (1941). Psychogenic episodes in the course of major psychoses. *J. Ment. Sci.*, **87**, 383-389

Armbrustmacher, V.W. (1979). Pathology of dementia. *Pathol. Ann.*, **14** (1) 145-173

Barette, J. and Marsden, C.D. (1979). Attitudes of families to some aspects of Huntington's chorea. *Psychol. Med.*, **9**, 327-336

Barron, S.A., Jacobs, L. and Kinkel, W.R. (1976). Changes in size of normal lateral ventricles during ageing determined by computerised tomography. *Neurology*, **26**, 1011-1013

Behan, P.O. and Behan, W.M.H. (1979). Possible immunological factors in Alzheimer's disease. In Glen, A.J.M. and Whalley, L.J. (eds). *Alzheimer's Disease: Early Recognition of Potentially Reversible Deficits*. (Edinburgh: Churchill Livingstone)

Benson, D.F. (1975). The hydrocephalic dementias. In Benson, D.F. and Blumer, D. (eds). *Psychiatric Aspects of Neurological Disease*. (New York: Grune and Stratton)

Bentson, N., Larsen, B. and Lassen, N. (1975). Chronically impaired autoregulation of cerebral blood flow in long-term diabetics. *Stroke*, **6**, 497-502

Berger, H. (1932). In Hans Berger on the Electroencephalogram in Man. (Tr. and ed. P. Gloor (1969) *Electroenceph. Clin. Neurophysiol.*, Suppl. **28**,151-171

Bergmann, K. (1979). The problem of early diagnosis. In Glen, A.J.M. and Whalley, L.J. (eds). *Alzheimer's Disease; Early Recognition of Potentially Reversible Deficits*. (Edinburgh: Churchill Linvingstone)

Bergmann, K., Kay, D.W.K., McKechnie, A.A., Foster, E. and Roth, M. (1971). A follow-up study of randomly selected community residents to assess the effects of chronic brain syndrome and cerebrovascular disease. *Excerpta Medica International Congress Series No. 274*, Psychiatry II, 856-865

Bergmann, K., Foster, E.M., Justice, A.W. and Matthews, V. (1978). Management of the demented elderly patient in the community. *Br. J. Psychiatry.*, **132**, 441-449

Besson, J.A.O., Corrigan, F.M., Foreman, E.I., Ashcroft, G.W. Eastwood, L.M. and Smith, F.W. (1983). Differentiating senile dementia of Alzheimer type and multi-infarct dementia by proton NMR imaging *Lancet*, **2**, 789

Binswanger, O. (1894). Die Abrunzung der allgeimeinen progressiven paralyse. *Berl. Klin. Wochenschr.*, **31**, 1103-1105, 1137-1139, 1180-1186

Bird, T.D., Stranahan, S., Sumi, S.M. and Raskind, M. (1983). Alzheimer's disease: choline acetyl-transferase activity in brain tissue from clinical and pathological subgroups. *Ann. Neurol.*, **14**, 284-293

Birkett, D.P. (1972). The psychiatric differentiation of senility and arteriosclerosis. *Br. J. Psychiatry*, **120**, 321-325

Blackburn, I.M. (1979). Problems of measurement in Alzheimer's disease. In Glen, A.I.M. and Whalley, L.J. (eds). *Alzheimer's Disease: Early Recognition of Potentially Reversible Deficits.* (Edinburgh: Churchill Livingstone)

Blane, D. (1982). Elderly people and health. In Patrick, D.L. and Scrambler, G. (eds). *Sociology as Applied to Medicine.* (London: Baillière Tindall)

Bondareff, W., Baldy, R. and Levy, R. (1981). Quantitative computed tomography in senile dementia. *Arch. Gen. Psychiatry*, **38**, 1365-1368

Bowen, D.M. (1981). Alzheimer's disease. In Davison, A.N. and Thompson, R.H.S. (eds). *The Molecular Basis of Neuropathology.* (London: Edward Arnold)

Bowen, D.M., Smith, C.B., White, P. and Davison, A.N. (1976). Neurotransmitter-related enzymes and indices of hypoxia in senile dementia and other abiotrophies. *Brain*, **99**, 459-496

Bowen, D.M. and Davison, A.N. (1978). Biochemical changes in the normal ageing brain and in dementia. In Isaacs, B. (ed). *Recent Advances in Geriatric Medicine.* (Edinburgh: Churchill Livingstone)

Bowen, D.M. and Davison, A.N. (1981). The neurochemistry of ageing and senile dementia. In Matthews, W.B. and Glaser, G.H. (eds). *Recent Advances in Clinical Neurology.* Vol. 3. (Edinburgh: Churchill Livingstone)

Bowen, D.M., Sims, N.R., Davison, A.N., Neary, D. and Thomas, D.J. (1981). Acetylcholine synthesis in control and dementia brain tissue. In Rose, F.C. (ed).*Metabolic Disorders of the Nervous System.* (London: Pitman)

Bowen, D.M., Allen, S.J., Benton, J.S., Goodhardt, M.J., Haan, E.A., Palmer, A.M., Sims, N.R., Smith, C.C.T., Spillane, J.A., Esiri, M.M., Neary, D., Snowdon, J.S., Wilcock, G.K. and Davison, A.N. (1983). Biochemical assessment of serotonergic and cholinergic dysfunction and cerebral atrophy in Alzheimer's disease. *J. Neurochem.*, **41**, 266-272

Brain, W.R. and Henson, R.A. (1958). Neurological syndromes associated with carcinoma. *Lancet*, **2**, 971-975

Branconnier, R. and Cole. J.O. (1977a). Senile dementia and drug therapy. In Nandy, K. and Sherwin, I. (eds). *The Ageing Brain and Senile Dementia.* (New York: Plenum Press)

Branconnier, R. and Cole, J.O. (1977b). Effects of chronic papaverine administration on mild senile organic brain syndrome. *J. Am. Geriat. Soc.*, **25**, 458-462

Burnet, F.M. (1981). A possible role of zinc in the pathology of dementia. *Lancet*, **1**, 186-188

Busse, E.W., Barnes, R.H., Friedman, E.L. and Kelty, E.J. (1956). Psychological functioning of aged individuals with normal and abnormal electroencephalograms. *J. Nerv. Ment. Dis.*, **124**, 135-141

Caine, E. (1981). Pseudodementia: current concepts and future directions *Arch. Gen. Psychiatry*, **38**, 1359-1364

Caplan, L. (1979). Chronic vascular dementia. *Primary Care*, **6**, (4) 843-848

Caplan, L. and Schoene, W. (1978). Clinical features of subcortical arteriosclerotic encephalopathy (Binswanger's disease). *Neurology*, **28**, 1206

Claveria, L.E., Moseley, I.F. and Stevenson, J.F. (1977). The clinical significance of cerebral atrophy as shown by CAT. In Du Boulay, G.H. and Mosele, I.F. (eds). *Computerised axial tomography in clinical practice.* (New York: Springer Verlag)

Cloe, L.E. (1976). Health planning for computer tomography: perspectives and problems. *Amer. J. Roentgenol.*, **127**, 187

COMBAT (1982). *Huntington's Chorea.* A booklet for family doctors and other professionals. (Association to Combat Huntington's Chorea)

Constantinidis, J., Krassoievitch, M. and Tissot, R. (1969). Correlations entre les perturbations electro-encephalographiques et les lesions anatomo-histologiques dans les demences. *Encephale*, **58**, 19-52 (quoted by Obrist, 1978)

Copeland, J.R.M., Kelleher, M.J., Kellett, J.M., Gourlay, A.J., Gurland, B.J., Fleiss, J.L. and Sharpe, L. (1976). A semi-structured clinical interview for the assessment of diagnosis and mental state in the elderly: the Geriatric Mental State Schedule I. Development and reliability. *Psychol. Med.*,6, 439-449

Corsellis, J.A.N. (1969). The pathology of dementia. *Br. J. Hosp. Med.*, 2, 695

Corsellis, J.A.N. (1978). Post-traumatic dementia. In Katzman, R., Terry, R.D. and Bick, K.L. (eds). *Alzheimer's Disease: Senile Dementia and Related Disorders*. (New York: Raven Press)

Corsellis, J.A.N. (1979). On the transmission of dementia. A personal view of the slow virus problem. *Br. J. Psychiatry*, 134, 553-559

Corsellis, J.A.N., Bruton, C.J. and Freeman-Browne, D. (1973). The aftermath of boxing. *Psychol. Med.*, 3, 270-303

Crapper, D.R., Karlik, S. and De Boni, U. (1978). Aluminum and other metals in senile (Alzheimer) dementia. In Katzman, R., Terry, R.D. and Bick, K.L. (eds). *Alzheimer's Disease: Senile Dementia and Related Disorders*. (New York: Raven Press)

Creutzfeldt, H.G. (1920). Uber eine eigenartige herdformige Erkrankung des Zentral nervensystems. *Z. Neurol. Pyschiatry*, 57, 1-18

Crow, T.J. (1981). Biochemical aspects of memory. In Rose, F.C. (ed.). *Metabolic Disorders of the Nervous System*. (London: Pitman Medical)

Cutting, J. (1978). The relationship between Korsakov's syndrome and 'alcoholic dementia'. *Br. J. Psychiatry*, 132, 240-251

Dewhurst, K. (1969). The neurosyphilitic psychoses of today. A survey of 91 cases. *Br. J. Psychiatry*, 115, 31-38

Diesenhammer, E. and Jellinger, K. (1974). EEG in senile dementia. *Electroenceph. Clin. Neurophysiol.*, 36, 91

Donaldson, A.A. (1979). CT scan in Alzheimer pre-senile dementia. In Glen, A.I.M. and Whalley, L.J. (eds). *Alzheimer's Disease: Early Recognition of Potentially Reversible Deficits*. (Edinburgh: Churchill Livingstone)

Du Boulay, G.H., Bull, J.W.D., Gawler, J. and Marshall, J. (1975). Computerised tomography. An evaluation in patients with dementia. *International Symposium on Computed Tomography, Bermuda.*

Eisdorfer, C. and Keckich, W. (1980). The normal psychopathology of ageing. In Cole, J.O. and Barrett, J.E. (eds). *Psychopathology in the Aged*. (New York: Raven Press)

Esquirol, J.E.D. (1838). *Traite des Maladies Mentales*. (Paris)

Feinberg, I., Koresko, R.L. and Heller, N. (1967). EEG sleep patterns as a function of normal and pathological ageing in man. *J. Psychiatr. Res.*, 5, 107-144

Filskov, S.B. and Goldstein, S.G. (1974). Diagnostic validity of the Halstead-Reitan neuropsychological battery. *J. Consult. Clin. Psychol.*, 42, 382-388

Fisher, C.M. (1965). Lacunes. Small deep cerebral infarcts. *Neurology*, 15, 774

Fisher, J. and Gonda, T.A. (1955). Neurologic techniques and Rorschach test in detecting brain pathology. A study of comparative validities. *Arch. Neurol.*, 74, 117-124

Folstein, M.F. and McHugh, P.R. (1978). Dementia syndrome of depression. In Katzman, R., Terry, R.D. and Bick, K.L. (eds). *Alzheimer's Disease: Senile Dementia and Related Disorders*. (New York: Raven Press)

Fox, J.H., Topel, J.L. and Huckman, M.S. (1975). Use of computerised axial tomography in senile dementia. *J. Neurol. Neurosurg. Psychiatry*, 38, 948-953

Frackowiak, R.S.J., Lenzi, G.L., Jones, T. and Heather, J.D. (1980). Quantitative measurement of regional cerebral blood flow and oxygen metabolism in man using Oxygen-15 and positron emission tomography: theory, procedure and normal values. *J. Comp. Assist. Tomography*, 4, 727-736

Frackowiak, R.S.J., Pozzilli, C., Legg, N.J., Du Boulay, G.H., Marshall, J., Lenzi, G.L. and Jones, T. (1981). Regional cerebral oxygen supply and utilisation in dementia. *Brain*, 104, 753-778

Gajdusek, D.C. and Zigas, V. (1957). Degenerative disease of the central nervous system in New Guinea. The endemic occurrence of 'Kuru' in the native population. *N. Engl. J. Med.*, 257 (30), 974-978

Ganser, S.J.M. (1898). A peculiar hysterical state. *Arch. Psychiat. NervKrankh.*, 30, 633-40 (Tr. C.E. Schorer (1965). *Br. J. Criminol.*, 5, 120-126)

Gascon, G.G. and Gilles, F. (1973). Limbic dementia. *J. Neurol, Neurosurg. Psychiatry* 36, 421-430

Gawler, J. (1981). Computed axial tomography of the brain. In Dawson, A.M., Besser, G.M.

and Compston, N. (eds). *Recent Advances in Medicine* Vol 18. (Edinburgh: Churchill Livingstone)

Gawler, J., Du Boulay, G.H., Bull, J.W.D. and Marshall, J. (1976). Computerised tomography (EMI scanner): a comparison with pneumencephalography and ventriculography. *J. Neurol. Neurosurg. Psychiatry*, **39**, 203-211

George, A.E., de Leon, M.J., Ferris, S.H. and Kricheff, I.I. (1981). Parenchymal CT correlates of senile dementia (Alzheimer Disease): loss of gray-white matter discriminability. *Am. J. Neuroradiol.*, **2**, 205-213

Gibson, A.J., Moyes, I.C.A. and Kendrick, D. (1980). Cognitive assessement of the elderly long-stay patient. *Br. J. Psychiatry*, **137**, 551-557

Glen, A.I.M. and Christie, J.E. (1979). Early diagnosis of Alzheimer's disease: working definitions for clinical and laboratory criteria. In Glen, A.I.M. and Whalley, L.J. (eds). *Alzheimer's Disease; Early Recognition of Potentially Reversible Deficits.* (Edinburgh: Churchill Livingstone)

Golden, C.J., Osmon, D.C., Moses, J.A. and Berg, R.A. (1981). *Interpretation of the Halstead–Reitan Neuropsychological Test Battery.* (New York: Grune and Stratton)

Gonzalez, C.F., Lantiert, R.L. and Nathan, R.J. (1978). The CT scan appearance of the brain in the normal elderly population: a correlative study. *Neuroradiology*, **16**, 120-122

Griesinger, W. (1845). *Pathologie und Therapie der Psychischen Krankheiten.* (Tr. C.L. Robertson, 1862. London: New Sydenham Society)

Growdon, J.H. and Corkin, S. (1980). Neurochemical approaches to the treatment of senile dementia. In Cole, J.O. and Barrett, J.E. (eds). *Psychopathology in the Aged.* (New York: Raven Press)

Gurland, B.J., Fleiss, J.L., Goldberg, K., Sharpe, L., Copeland, J.R.M., Kelleher, M.J. and Kellett, J.M. (1976). A semi-structured clinical interview for the assessment of diagnosis and mental state in the elderly: the Geriatric Mental State Schedule. II. A factor analysis. *Psychol. Med.*, **6**, 451-459

Gustafson, L. (1979). Regional cerebral blood flow in Alzheimer's disease – differential diagnosis, the possibility of early recognition and evaluation of treatment. In Glen, A.I.M. and Whalley, L.J. (eds). *Alzheimer's Disease: Early Recognition of Potentially Reversible Deficits.* (Edinburgh: Churchill Livingstone)

Gustafson, L. and Hagberg, B. (1978). Recovery in hydrocephalic dementia after shunt operation. *J. Neurol. Neurosurg. Psychiatry*, **41**, 940-947

Gustafson, L., Hagberg, B. and Ingvar, D.H. (1978). Speech disturbances in presenile dementia related to local cerebral blood flow abnormalities in the dominant hemisphere. *Brain Lang.*, **5**, 103-118

Gyldensted, C. (1977). Measurements of the normal ventricular system and hemispheric sulci of 100 adults with computed tomography. *Neuroradiology*, **14**, 183-192

Hachinski, V.C., Lassen, N.A. and Marshall, J. (1974). Multi-infarct dementia. *Lancet*, **2**, 207-209

Hachinski, V.C., Iliff, L.D., Zilkha, E., Du Boulay, G.H., McAllister, V.L., Marshall, J., Ross Russell, R.W. and Symon, L. (1975). Cerebral blood flow in dementia. *Arch. Neurol,*, **32**, 632-637

Hachinski, V.C. (1978). Cerebral blood flow: differentiation of Alzheimer's Disease from multi-infarct dementia. In Katzman, R., Terry, R.D. and Bick, K.L. (eds). *Alzheimer's Disease: Senile Dementia and Related Disorders.* (New York: Raven Press)

Hadlow, W.J. (1959). Scrapie and Kuru. *Lancet*, **2**, 289-290

Hagberg, B. (1978). Defects of immediate memory related to cerebral blood flow distribution (quoted by Ingvar *et al*, 1978)

Hagberg, B. and Ingvar, D.H. (1976). Cognitive reduction in presenile dementia related to regional abnormalities of the cerebral blood flow. *Br. J. Psychiatry*, **128**, 209-222

Hakim, S. and Adams, R.D. (1965). The special clinical problem of symptomatic hydrocephalus with normal cerebrospinal fluid pressure: observations on cerebrospinal fluid hydrodynamics. *J. Neurol. Sci.*, **2**, 307-327

Hare, E.H. (1959). The origin and spread of dementia paralytica. *J. Ment. Sci.*, **105**, 594-626

Hare, E.H. (1974). The changing content of psychiatric illness. *J. Psychosom. Res.*, **18**, 283-289

Harner, R.N. (1975). EEG evaluation of the patient with dementia. In Benson, D.F. and Blumer, D. (eds) *Psychiatric Aspects of Neurological Disease.* (New York: Grune and Stratton)

Harrison, M.J.G., Thomas, D.J., Du Boulay, G.H. and Marshall, J. (1979). Multi-infarct dementia. *J. Neurol. Sci.*, **40**, 97-103

Haslam, J. (1798). *Observations on Insanity.* (London)

Hedlund, S., Kohler, V., Nylin, G., Olsson, R., Regustrom, V., Rothstrom, E. and Astrom, K.E. (1964). Cerebral blood circulation in dementia. *Acta. Psychiatr. Scand.*, **40**, 77-106

Henry, G.W. (1941). Organic mental diseases. In Zilboorg, G. and Henry, G.W. (eds). *A History of Medical Psychology.* (New York: W.W. Norton and Co)

Henson, R.A. and Urich, H. (1982). *Cancer and the Nervous System.* (London: Blackwell Scientific Publications)

Heyman, A. (1978). Differentiation of Alzheimer's Disease from multi-infarct dementia. In Katzman, R., Terry, R.D. and Bick, K.L. (eds). *Alzheimer's Disease: Senile Dementia and Related Disorders.* (New York: Raven Press)

Hodkinson, H.M. (1973). Mental impairment in the elderly. *J. Roy. Coll. Phys, Lond.*, **7**, 305-317

Hughes, C.P., (1978). The differential diagnosis of dementia in the senium. In Nandy, K. (ed.). *Senile Dementia: A Biomedical Approach.* (Amsterdam: Elsevier North-Holland Biomedical Press)

Hughes, J.R., Williams, J.G. and Currier, R.D. (1976). An ergot alkaloid preparation (hydrergine) in the treatment of dementia: critical review of the clinical literature. *J. Am. Geriatr. Soc.*, **24**, 490-497

Hunter, R.A. and Macalpine, I. (1963). *Three Hundred Years of Psychiatry, 1535-1860.* (London: Oxford University Press)

Huntington, G. (1872). On chorea. *Med. Surg. Rep.*, **26**, 317-321

Ingelfinger, F.J. (1980). Arrogance. *N. Engl. J. Med.*, **303**, 1507-1511

Ingvar, D.H. (1979). Hyperfrontal distribution of the grey matter blood flow in the resting conscious state (quoted in Ingvar, 1980)

Ingvar, D.H., (1980). Regional cerebral blood flow and psychopathology. In *Psychopathology in the Aged.* Ed. J.O. Cole and J.E. Barrett. (New York: Raven Press)

Ingvar, D.H. and Risberg, J. (1965). Influence of mental activity upon regional cerebral blood flow in man. *Acta Neurol. Scand.*, **41**, (suppl. 14), 93-96

Ingvar, D.H. and Risberg, J. (1967). Increase of regional cerebral blood flow during mental effort in normals and in patients with focal brain disorders. *Exp. Brain Res.*, **3**, 195-211

Ingvar, D.H. and Schwartz, M.S. (1974). Blood flow patterns induced in the dominant hemisphere by speech and reading. *Brain*, **96**, 274-288

Ingvar, D.H., Risberg, J. and Schwartz, M.S. (1975). Evidence of subnormal function of association cortex in presenile dementia. *Neurology*, **10**, 964-974

Ingvar, D.H., Brun, A., Hagberg, B. and Gustafson, L. (1978). Regional cerebral blood flow in the dominant hemisphere in confirmed cases of Alzheimer's disease, Pick's disease and multi-infarct dementia: relationship to clinical symptomatology and neuropathological findings. In Katzman, R., Terry, R.D. and Bick, K.L. (eds). *Alzheimer's Disease: Senile Dementia and Related Disorders.* (New York: Raven Press)

Jacobs, L., Kinkel, W.R. and Heffner, R.R. (1976). Autopsy correlations of computerised tomography; experience with 6000 CT scans. *Neurology* (Minneap.), **26**, 1111-1118

Jacoby, R.J. (1982). Computed tomography in dementia and depression. In Granville-Grossman, K. (ed.) *Recent Advances in Clinical Psychiatry.* Vol 4. (Edinburgh: Churchill Livingstone)

Jacoby, R.J., Levy, R. and Dawson, J.M. (1980). Computed tomography in the elderly: 1. The normal population. *Br. J. Psychiatry*, **136**, 249-255

Jacoby, R.J. and Levy, R. (1980). Computed tomography in the elderly: 2. Senile dementia: diagnosis and functional impairment. *Br. J. Psychiatry*, **136**, 256-269

Jakob, A. (1921). Uber eigenartige Erkrankung des Zentralnerven systems mit bemerkenswertem anatomischen Befunde (Spastische Pseudosklerose-Encephalomyelopathie mit dissemimerten Degenerationsherden). *Deutsche Z. Nerveheilkunde*, **70**, 132-146

Jellinger, K. (1976). Neuropathological aspects of dementias resulting from abnormal blood and cerebrospinal fluid dynamics. *Acta Neurol.* (Belg.), **76**, 83-102

Jervis, G.A. (1948). Early senile dementia in mongoloid idiocy. *Am. J. Psychiatry*, **105**, 102-106

Jervis, G.A. and Soltz, S.E. (1936). Alzheimer's disease – the so-called juvenile type. *Am. J. Psychiatry*, **93**, 39-56

Johannesson, G., Brun, A., Gustafson, I. and Ingvar, D.H. (1977). EEG in presenile dementia related to cerebral blood flow and autopsy findings. *Acta. Neurol. Scand.*, **56**, 89-103

Kaneko, Z. (1969). *Abstract of the Proceedings of the 8th International Congress of Gerontology, Washington D.C.* (quoted in Royal College of Physicians, 1981)

Kaszniak, A.W., Fox, J., Gandell, D.L., Garron, D.C., Huckman, M.S. and Ramsey, R.G. (1978). Predictors of mortality in presenile and senile dementia. *Ann. Neurol,*, **3**, 246-252

Katzman, R. (1976). Cerebrospinal fluid physiology and normal pressure hydrocephalus. In Gershon, S. and Terry, R.D. (eds). *Neurobiology of Ageing.* (New York: Raven Press)

Katzman, R. (1977). Normal pressure hydrocephalus. In Wells, C.E. (ed.). *Dementia.* (Philadelphia: Davis)

Katzman, R. (1978). Normal pressure hydrocephalus. In Katzman, R., Terry, R.D. and Bick, K.L. (eds). *Alzheimer's Disease: Senile Dementia and Related Disorders.* (New York: Raven Press)

Kay, D.W.K. (1962). Outcome and cause of death in mental disorders of old age: a long-term followup of functional and organic psychoses. *Acta Psychiat. Scand.*, **38**, 249-276

Kay, D.W.K. (1972). In Gaitz, C.M. (ed.). *Ageing and the Brain* (quoted by Roth, 1979)

Kay, D.W.K., Beamish, P. and Roth, M. (1964). Old age mental disorders in Newcastle-upon Tyne I. A study of prevalence. *Br. J. Psychiatry*, **110**, 146-158

Kay, D.W.K., Bergmann, K., Foster, E.M., McKechnie, A.A. and Roth, M. (1970). Mental illness and hospital usage in the elderly: a random sample followed up. *Compr. Psychiatry*, **1**, 26-35

Kendell, R. (1974). The stability of psychiatric diagnosis. *Br. J. Psychiatry*, **124**, 352-356

Kendell, R. (1975). Schizophrenia: the remedy for diagnostic confusion. In Silverstone, T. and Barraclough, B. (eds). *Contemporary Psychiatry.* (London: Royal College of Psychiatrists)

Kety, S.S. (1967). The central physiological and pharmacological effects of the biogenic amines and their correlations with behaviour. In Quinton, G.C., Melneckich, T. and Schmidt, F. (eds). *The Neurosciences.* (New York: Rockefeller University Press)

Kety, S.S. (1972). The double role of the adrenergic systems of the cortex in learning (quoted in Folstein and McHugh, 1978)

Kety, S.S. and Schmidt, C.F. (1945). The determination of cerebral blood flow in man by the use of nitrous oxide in low concentrations. *Am. J. Physiol.*, **143**, 53

Kidd, C.B. (1962). Criteria for admission of the elderly to geriatric and psychiatric units. *J. Ment.Sci.*, **108**, 68-74

Kinkel, W.R. and Jacobs, L. (1976). Computerised axial transverse tomography in cerebrovascular disease, *Neurology* (Minneap.), **26**, 924-930

Kral, V.A. (1962). Senescent fortgetfulness: Benign and malignant. *Can. Med. Assoc. J.*, **86**, 257-260

Kral, V.A. (1978). Benign senescent forgetfulness. In Katzman, R., Terry, R.D. and Bick, K.L. (eds). *Alzheimer's Disease: Senile Dementia and Related Disorders.* (New York: Raven Press)

Kugler, J., Oswald, W.D., Herzfeld, U., Sens, R., Pingel, J. and Welzel, D. (1978). Long-term treatment of the symptoms of senile cerebral insufficiency: a prospective study of hydrergine (quoted in Reisberg *et al.*, 1980)

Ladurner, G., Iliff, L.D., Sager, W.D. and Lechner, H. (1982). A clinical approach to vascular (multi-infarct) dementia. In Hoyer, S. (ed.). *The Aging Brain.* (Berlin: Springer-Verlag)

Larsson, T., Sjogren, T. and Jacobsen, G. (1963). Senile dementia. *Acta Psychiat. Scand.*, **39** (suppl. 167)

Lassen, N.A. and Ingvar, D.H. (1972). Radioisotopic assessment of regional cerebral blood flow. *Prog. Nucl. Med.*, **1**. 376-409

Lawton, M.P. (1980). Psychosocial and environmental approaches to the care of senile dementia patients. In Cole, J.O. and Barrett, J.E. (eds). *Psychopathology in the Aged.* (New York: Raven Press)

Lenzi, G.L., Jones, T., Moss, S. and Thomas, D.J. (1977). The relationship between regional oxygen utilization and cerebral blood flow in multi-infarct dementia. *Acta Neurol. Scand.*, Suppl. **56** (64), 248-249

208

Libow, L.S. (1978). Epidemiology – excess mortality and proximate causes of death. In Katzman, R., Terry, R.D. and Bick, K.L. (eds). *Alzheimer's Disease: Senile Dementia and Related Disorders*. (New York: Raven Press)

Lishman, W.A. (1978). *Organic Psychiatry*. (London: Blackwell Scientific Publications)

Lishman, W.A. (1981). Cerebral disorder in alcoholism. *Brain*, **104**, 1-20

Locker, D. (1982). The family and illness. In Patrick, D.L. and Scrambler, G. (eds). *Sociology as Applied to Medicine*. (London, Ballière Tindall)

Loizou, L.A., Kendall, B.E. and Marshall, J. (1981). Subcortical arteriosclerotic encephalopathy: a clinical and radiological investigation. *J. Neurol. Neurosurg. Psychiatry*, **44**, 294-304

Maggs, R. and Turton, E.C. (1956). Some EEG findings in old age and their relationship to affective disorder. *J. Ment. Sci.*, **102**, 812-818

Mahendra, B. (1983). 'Pseudodementia': an illogical and misleading concept. *Br. J. Psychiatry*, **143**, 202

Mahendra, B. (1984). Dementia and the abnormal dexamethasone suppression test. *Br. J. Psychiatry*, **144**, 98-99

Mann, D.M.A., Yates, P.O., Bansal, D.V. and Marshall, D.J. (1981). Hypothalamus and dementia. *Lancet*, **1**, 393-394

Mann, D.M.A. and Yates, P.O. (1982). Ageing, nucleic acids and pigments. In Smith, W.T. and Cavanagh, J.B. (eds). *Recent Advances in Neuropathology*. Vol 2. (Edinburgh: Churchill Livingstone)

Mann, D.M.A., Yates, P.O. and Hawkes, J. (1982). The noradrenergic system in Alzheimer and multi-infarct dementias. *J. Neurol. Neurosurg. Psychiatry*, **45**, 113-119

Mann, D.M.A., Yates, P.O. and Marcyniuk, B. (1984). A comparison of changes in the nucleus basalis and locus caeruleus in Alzheimer's disease. *J. Neurol. Neurosurg. Psychiatry*, **47**, 201-203

Marcer, D. (1979). Measuring memory change in Alzheimer's disease. In Glen, A.I.M. and Whalley, L.J. (eds). *Alzheimer's Disease: Early Recognition of Potentially Reversible Deficits*. (Edinburgh: Churchill Livingstone)

Marcus, A.J. (1977). Aspirin and thromboembolism – a possible dilemma. *N. Engl. J. Med.*, **297**, 1284-1285

Marsden, C.D. (1982). Basal ganglia disease. *Lancet*, **2**, 1141-1147

Marsden, C.D. and Harrison, M.J.G. (1972). Outcome of investigation of patients with presenile dementia. *Br. Med. J.*, **2**, 249-252

Martland, H.S. (1928). Punch drunk. *J. Am. Med. Assoc.*, **91**, 1103-1107

Masters, C.L., Harris, J.O., Gajdusek, D.C., Gibbs, C.J., Bernoulli, C. and Asher, D.M. (1979). Creutzfeldt-Jakob disease: patterns of worldwide occurrence and significance of familial and sporadic clustering. *Ann. Neurol.*, **5**, 177-188

Masters, C.L. and Gajdusek, D.C. (1982). The spectrum of Creutzfeldt-Jakob disease and the virus-induced subacute spongiform encephalopathies. In Smith, W.T. and Cavanagh, J.B. (eds). *Recent Advances in Neuropathology*, Vol 2. (Edinburgh: Churchill Livingstone)

Mayer-Gross, W., Slater, E. and Roth, M. (1960). *Clinical Psychiatry*, 2nd edn. (London: Cassell)

Mayeux, R., Stern, Y., Rosen, J. and Benson, D.F. (1983). Is 'subcortical dementia' a recognizable clinical entity? *Ann. Neurol.*, **14**, 278-283

McAllister, T.W. (1983). Pseudodementia. *Am. J. Psychiatry,* **140**, 528-533

McAllister, T.W. and Price, T.R.P. (1982). Severe depressive pseudodementia with and without dementia. *Am. J. Psychiatry*, **139**, 626-629

McAllister, T.W., Ferrell, R.B., Price, T.R.P. and Neville, M.B. (1982) The dexamethasone suppression test in two patients with severe depressive pseudodementia. *Am. J. Psychiatry*, **139**, 479-481

McQuillan, I.M., Lopec, C.A. and Vibal, J.R. (1974). Evaluation of EEG and clinical changes associated with Parabid therapy in chronic brain syndrome. *Curr. Ther. Res.*, **16**, 49-58

Melamed, E., Lavy, S., Siew, F., Bentin, S. and Cooper, G. (1978). Correlation between regional cerebral blood flow and brain atrophy in dementia. *J. Neurol. Neurosurg. Psychiatry*, **41**, 894-899

Millard, P.H. (1981). Last scene of all. *Br. Med. J.*, **4**, 1559-1560

Miller, E. (1977). *Abnormal Ageing*. (London: Wiley)

Mindham, R.H.S., Ahmed, S.W.A. and Clough, C.G. (1982). A controlled study of dementia in Parkinson's disease. *J. Neurol. Neurosurg. Psychiatry*, **45**, 969-974

Mohr, J.P. (1978). Transient ischaemic attacks and the prevention of strokes. Editorial, *N. Engl. J. Med.*, 299, 2, 93-95

Muller, H.F. (1978). The electroencephalogram in senile dementia. In Nandy, K. (ed.), *Senile Dementia: A Biomedical Approach*. (Amsterdam: Elsevier North-Holland Biomedical Press)

Naeser, M.A., Gebhardt, C. and Levine, H.L. (1980). Decreased computerised tomography numbers in patients with presenile dementia. *Arch. Neurol.*, 37, 401-409

Naguib, M. and Levy, R. (1982). Prediction of outcome in senile dementia – a computed tomography study. *Br. J. Psychiatry*, **140**, 263-267

Nielson, J. (1962). Quoted in Report of Royal College of Physicians, 1981

Nott, P.N. and Fleminger, J.J. (1975). Presenile dementia. The difficulties of early diagnosis. *Acta Psychiat. Scand.*, **51**, 210-217

O'Brien, M.D. and Mallett, B.L. (1970). Cerebral cortex perfusion rates in dementia. *J. Neurol. Neurosurg. Psychiatry*, 33, 497-500

Obrist, W.D. (1954). The electroencephalogram of normal aged adults. *Electroencephalogr. Clin. Neurophysiol.*, 6, 235-244

Obrist, W.D. (1978a). Electroencephalography in ageing and dementia. In Katzman, R., Terry, R.D. and Bick, K.L. (eds). *Alzheimer's Disease: Senile Dementia and Related Disorders*. (New York: Raven Press)

Obrist, W.D. (1978b). Non-invasive studies of cerebral blood flow in ageing and dementia. In Katzman, R., Terry, R.D. and Bick, K.L. (eds). *Alzheimer's Disease: Senile Dementia and Related Disorders*. (New York: Raven Press)

Obrist, W.D., Busse, E.W. and Henry, C.E. (1961). Relation of electroencephalogram to blood pressure in elderly persons. *Neurology* (Minneap.), **11**, 151-158

Obrist, W.D. and Busse, E.W. (1965). The electroencephalogram in old age. In Wilson, W.P. (ed.). *Applications of Electroencephalography in Psychiatry*. (Durham (USA): Duke University Press)

Obrist, W.D., Thompson, H.K. Jnr., Wang, H.S. and Wilkinson, W.E. (1975). Regional cerebral blood flow estimated by xenon-133 inhalation. *Stroke*, 6, 245-256

Office of Health Economics (1979). *Dementia in Old Age*. (London)

Office of Health Economics (1980). *Huntington's Chorea*. (London)

Oleson, J. (1971). Contralateral focal increase of cerebral blood flow in man during arm work. *Brain*, 94, 635-646

Oliver, J.E. (1970). Huntington's chorea in Northamptonshire. *Br. J. Psychiatry*, **116**, 241-253

Opit, L.J. (1977). Domiciliary care for the elderly sick - economy or neglect? *Br. Med. J.*, 1 30-33

Otomo, E. (1966). Electroencephalography in old age: dominant Alpha pattern. *Electroenceph. Clin. Neurophysiol.*, **21**, 489-491

Perez, F.I. (1980). Behavioural studies of dementia: methods of investigation and analysis. In Cole, J.O. and Barrett, J.E. (eds). *Psychopathology in the Aged*. (New York: Raven Press)

Perez, F.I., Rivera, V.M., Meyer, J.S., Gray, J.R.A., Taylor, R.L. and Mathew, N.T. (1975). Analysis of intellectual and cognitive performance in patients with multi-infarct dementia, vertebrobasilar insufficiency with dementia and Alzheimer's disease. *J. Neurol. Neurosurg. Psychiatry*, 38, 533-540

Perez, F.I., Stump, D.A., Gray, J.R.A. and Hart, V.R. (1976). Intellectual performance in multi-infarct dementia and Alzheimer's disease. A replication study. *Can. J. Neurol. Sci.*, 3, 181-187

Perez, F.I., Gray, J.R.A. and Cooke, N.A. (1978). Neuropsychological aspects of Alzheimer's disease and multi-infarct dementia. In Nandy, K. (ed.). *Senile Dementia: A Biomedical Approach*. (Amsterdam: Elsevier-North Holland Biomedical Press)

Perry, E.K. (1979). Correlations between psychiatric, neuropathological and biochemical findings in Alzheimer's disease. In Glen, A.I.M. and Whalley, L.J. (eds). *Alzheimer's Disease: Early Recognition of Potentially Reversible Deficits*. (Edinburgh: Churchill Livingstone)

Perry, E.K. and Perry, R.H. (1982). Neurotransmitter and neuropeptide systems in Alzheimer-type dementia. In Hoyer, S. (ed.). *The Aging Brain*. (Berlin: Springer-verlag)

Perry, R.H., Tomlinson, B.E., Candy, J.M., Blessed, G., Foster, J.F., Bloxham, C.A. and Perry, E.R. (1983). Cortical cholinergic deficit in mentally impaired Parkinsonian patients. *Lancet*, 2, 789-790

210

Perry, T.L. (1981). Some ethical problems in Huntington's chorea. *Can. Med. Assoc. J.*, **125**, 1098-1100

Perry, T.L., Wright, J.M., Hansen, S. and MacLeod, P.M. (1979). Isoniazid therapy of Huntington disease. *Neurology* (Minneap)., **29**, 370-375

Pick, A. (1892). On the relation of senile cerebral atrophy and aphasia. *Prag. Mediz. Wachenschrift.*, **17**, 165-167

Plum, F. (1978). Metabolic dementias. In Katzman, R., Terry, R.D. and Bick, K.L. (eds). *Alzheimer's Disease: Senile Dementia and Related Disorders*. (New York: Raven Press)

Prichard, J.C. (1835). *A Treatise on Insanity*. (London)

Radue, E.W., Du Boulay, G.H., Harrison, M.J.G. and Thomas, D.J. (1978). Comparison of angiographic and CT findings between patients with multi-infarct dementia and those with dementia due to primary neuronal degeneration. *Neuroradiology*, **16**, 113-115

Reisberg, B., Ferris, S.H. and Gershon, S. (1980). Pharmacotherapy of senile dementia. In Cole, J.O. and Barrett, J.E. (eds). *Psychopathology in the Aged*. (New York: Raven Press)

Report of the Royal College of Physicians (1981). Organic Mental Impairment in the Elderly. *J. Royal. Coll. Phys. Lond.*, **15**, (3), 141-167

Risberg, J. (1980). Regional cerebral blood flow measurements by 133-Xe-inhalation: methodology and applications in neuropsychology and psychiatry. *Brain Lang.*, **9**, 9-34

Roberts, A.H. (1969). *Brain Damage in Boxers. A study of the prevalence of traumatic encephalopathy among ex-boxers*. (London: Pitman)

Roberts, M.A. and Caird, F.I. (1976). Computerised tomography and intellectual impairment in the elderly *J. Neurol. Neurosurg. Psychiatry*, **39**, 986-989

Roberts, M.A., McGeorge, A.P. and Caird, F.I. (1976). Electroencephalography and computerised tomography in vascular and non-vascular dementia in old age. *J. Neurol. Neurosurg. Psychiatry*, **41**, 903-906

Robertson, E.E. (1978). Organic disorders. In Forrest, A.D., Affleck, J.W. and Zealley, A.K. (eds). *Companion to Psychiatric Studies*, 2nd edn. (Edinburgh: Churchill Livingstone)

Robertson, G.M. (1923). The discovery of general paralysis. *J. Ment. Sci.*, **69**, 1

Robinson, R.A. (1961). Problems of drug trials in elderly people. *Geront. Clin.*, **3**, 247-257

Ron, M.A., Toone, B.K., Garralda, M.E. and Lishman, W.A. (1979). Diagnostic accuracy in presenile dementia *Br. J. Psychiatry*, **134**, 161-168

Ropper, A.H. (1979). A rational approach to dementia. *Can. Med. Assoc. J.*, **1212**, 1175-1188

Rosen, G. (1961). Cross cultural and historical approaches. In Hoch, P.H. and Zubin, J. (eds). *Psychopathology of Ageing*. (New York: Grune and Stratton)

Rosenberg, C.E., Anderson, D.C., Mahowald, M.W. and Larson, D. (1982). Computed tomography and EEG in patients without focal neurologic findings. *Arch. Neurol.*, **39**, 291-292

Rossor, M.N. (1981). Parkinson's disease and Alzheimer's disease as disorders of the isodendritic core. *Br. Med. J.*, **283**, 1588-1590

Rossor, M.N., Emson, P.C., Iversen, L.L., Mountjoy, C.Q., Roth, Sir Martin, Hawthorn, J., Ang, V.T.Y., Jenkins, J.S. and Fahrenkrug, J. (1981). Neuropeptides in senile dementia of Alzheimer type: studies on somatostatin, vasoactive intestinal polypeptides and vasopressin. In Rose, F.C. (ed.), *Metabolic Disorders of the Nervous System*. (London: Pitman Medical)

Rossor, M.N., Garrett, N.J., Johnson, A.L., Mountjoy, C.Q., Roth, M. and Iversen, L.L. (1982). A post-mortem study of the cholinergic and GABA systems in senile dementia. *Brain*, **105**, 313-330

Rossor, M.N., Iversen, L.L., Reynolds, G.P., Mountjoy, C.Q. and Roth, M. (1984). Early and late onset types of Alzheimer's disease are neurochemically distinct. *Br. Med. J.*, (In press)

Roth, M. (1955). The natural history of mental disorders arising in the senium. *J. Ment. Sci.*, **101**, 281-301

Roth, M. (1978). Diagnosis of senile and related forms of dementia. In Katzman, R., Terry, R.D. and Bick, K.L. (eds). *Alzheimer's Disease: Senile Dementia and Related Disorders*. (New York: Raven Press)

Roth, M. (1980). Senile dementia and its borderlands. In Cole, J.O. and Barrett, J.E. (eds). *Psychopathology in the Aged*. (New York: Raven Press)

Roth, M. (1982). Perspectives in the diagnosis of senile and presenile dementia of Alzheimer type. In Sarner, M. (ed.). *Advanced Medicine*. Vol 18. (London: Royal College of Physicians and Pitman Medical)

211

Sainsbury, P. and Grad, J. (1966). Quoted in Office of Health Economics, 1966

Scheinberg, P. (1978). Multi-infarct dementia. In Katzman, R., Terry, R.D. and Bick, K.L. (eds). *Alzheimer's Disease: Senile Dementia and Related Disorders*. (New York: Raven Press)

Schoenberg, B.S. (1978). Neuroepidemiologic considerations in studies of Alzheimer's disease – senile dementia. In Katzman, R., Terry, R.D. and Bick, K.L. (eds). *Alzheimer's Disease: Senile Dementia and Related Disorders*. (New York: Raven Press)

Shaw, T. and Meyer, J.S. (1982). Ageing and cerebrovascular disease. In Meyer, J.S. and Shaw, T. (eds). *Diagnosis and Management of Stroke and TIAs*. (California: Addison-Wesley)

Shraberg, D. (1978). The myth of pseudodementia: depression and the aging brain. *Am. J. Psychiatry*, **135**, 601-603

Signoret, J.L., Whiteley, A. and Lhermitte, F. (1978). Influence of choline on amnesia in early Alzheimer's disease. *Lancet*, **2**, 837

Silfverskiold, P., Gustafson, L., Johanson, M. and Risberg, J. (1979). Regional cerebral blood flow related to the effect of electroconvulsive therapy in depression. In Obiols, J. *et al.* (eds). *Biological Psychiatry Today*. (Amsterdam: Elsevier-North Holland)

Sim, M., Turner, E. and Smith, W.T. (1966). Cerebral biopsy in the investigation of presenile dementia. I. Clinical aspects. *Br. J. Psychiatry*, **112**, 119-125

Simard, D., Oleson, J., Paulson, O.B., Lassen, N.A. and Skinhoj, E. (1971). Regional cerebral blood flow and its regulation in dementia. *Brain*, **94**, 273-288

Sjogren, T., Sjogren, H. and Lindgren, A.G.H. (1952). Morbus Alzheimer and morbus Pick: genetic, clinical and patho-anatomical study. *Acta Psychiatr. Neurol. Scand.* (Suppl. 82), 1-152.

Slater, E. and Roth, M. (1969). *Clinical Psychiatry*, 3rd edn. (London: Cassell)

Smith, C.M. and Swash, M. (1978). Possible biochemical basis of memory disorder in Alzheimer Disease. *Ann. Neurol.*, **3**, 471-473

Smith, J.S. and Kiloh, L.G. (1981). The investigation of dementia: results in 200 consecutive admissions. *Lancet*, **1**, 824-827

Soininen, H., Partanen, V.J., Helkala, EL. and Riekkinen, P.J. (1981). EEG findings in senile dementia and normal ageing (quoted in Soininen *et al.*, 1982)

Soininen, H., Puranen, M. and Riekkinen, P.J. (1982). Computed tomography findings in senile dementia and normal ageing. *J. Neurol. Neurosurg. Psychiatry*, **45**, 50-54

Sourander, P. and Sjogren, H. (1970). The concept of Alzheimer's disease and its clinical implications. In Wolstenholme, G.E.W. and O'Connor, M.E. (eds). *Alzheimer's Disease and Related Conditions*. (London: Churchill)

Spokes, E.G.S. (1978). Quoted in OHE (1980)

Stern, R. and Eldridge, R. (1975). Attitudes of patients and their relatives to Huntington's disease. *J. Med. Genet.*, **12**, 217-223

Striano, S., Vacca, G., Bilo, L. and Meo, R. (1981). The electroencephalogram in dementia. *Acta Neurol.* (Napoli), **36**, 727-737

Synek, V. and Reuben, J.R. (1976). The ventricular-brain ratio using planimetric measurement of EMI scans. *Br. J. Radiol.*, **49**, 233-237

Teltcher, B. and Polgar, S. (1981). Objective knowledge about Huntington's disease and attitudes towards predictive testing of persons at risk. *J. Med. Genet.*, **18**, 31-39

Terry, R.D. (1976). Dementia. A brief and selective review. *Arch. Neurol.*, **33**, 1-4

Terry, R.D. (1978). Ageing, senile dementia and Alzheimer's disease. In Katzman, R., Terry, R.D. and Bick, K.L. (eds). *Alzheimer's Disease: Senile Dementia and Related Disorders*. (New York: Raven Press)

Terry, R.D. and Wisniewski, H. (1973). Ultra-structure of senile dementia and of experimental analogs. In Gaitz, C. (ed.). *Ageing and the Brain*. (New York: Plenum Press)

Tomlinson, B.E. (1972). Morphological brain changes in non-demented old people. In van Praag, H.M. and Kalverboer, A.F. (eds). *Ageing of the Central Nervous System*. (New York: De Ervon F. Bohun)

Tomlinson, B.E. (1979). The ageing brain. In Smith, W.T. and Cavanagh, J.B. (eds). *Recent Advances in Neuropathology*. Vol. 1. (Edinburgh: Churchill Livingstone)

Tomlinson, B.E., Blessed, G. and Roth, M. (1968). Observations on the brains of non-demented old people. *J. Neurol. Sci.*, **7**, 331-356

Tomlinson, B.E., Blessed, G. and Roth, M. (1970). Observations on the brains of demented old people. *J. Neurol. Sci.*, **1**, 205-242

REFERENCES

Tomlinson, B.E. and Henderson, G. (1976). Some quantitative cerebral findings in normal and demented old people. In Terry, R.D. and Gershon, S. (eds). *Neurobiology of Ageing*, Vol. 3. (New York: Raven Press)

Torack R.M. (1979). Adult dementia: history, biopsy, pathology. *Neurosurgery*, **4** (5), 434-442

Tyler, A. (1979). Quoted in OHE (1980)

Van Praag, H.M. (1977). Psychotropic drugs in the aged. *Compr. Psychiatry*, **18**, 429-442

Veall, N. and Mallett, B.L. (1966). Regional cerebral blood flow determination by Xenon-133 inhalation and external recording: The effect of arterial recirculation. *Clin. Sci.*, **30**, 353-369

Victor, M. and Banker, B.Q. (1978). Alcohol and dementia. In Katzman, R., Terry, R.D. and Bick, K.L. (eds). *Alzheimer's Disease: Senile Dementia and Related Disorders*. (New York: Raven Press)

Walker, N. (1968). *Crime and Insanity in England*. Vol. 1. (Edinburgh: Edinburgh University Press)

Walsh, A.C., Walsh, B.H. and Maloney, C. (1978). Senile–presenile dementia: follow-up data on an effective psychotherapy-anticoagulant regimen. *J. Am. Geriat. Soc.*, **26**, 467-470

Wang, H.S. (1978). Prognosis in dementia and related disorders in the aged. In Katzman, R., Terry, R.D. and Bick, K.L. (eds). *Alzheimer's Disease: Senile Dementia and Related Disorders*. (New York: Raven Press)

Wang, H.S. and Busse, E.W. (1975). Correlates of regional cerebral blood flow in elderly community residents. In Harper, A.M. *et al.* (eds). *Blood Flow and Metabolism in the Brain*. (Edinburgh: Churchill Livingstone)

Wells, C.E. (1979). Pseudodementia. *Am. J. Psychiatry*, **136** (7), 895-900.

Wells, C.E. (1980). The differential diagnosis of psychiatric disorders in the elderly. In Cole, J.O. and Barrett, J.E. (eds). *Psychopathology in the Aged*. (New York: Raven Press)

West, D.J. (1965). *Murder Followed By Suicide*. (London: Heinemann)

Whisnant, J.P. (1977). Indications for medical and surgical therapy for ischaemic stroke. *Adv. Neurol.*, **16**, 133-144

Will, R.G. and Matthews, W.B. (1984). A retrospective study of Creutzfeldt–Jakob disease in England and Wales 1970-79. I: Clinical features. *J. Neurol. Neurosurg. Psychiatry*, **47**, 134-140

Wolf, P.A. and Kannel, W.A. (1982). Controllable risk factors for stroke: preventive implications of trends in stroke mortality. In Meyer, J.S. and Shaw, T. (eds). *Diagnosis and Management of Stroke and TIAs*. (California: Addison-Wesley)

World Health Organization (1972). *Psychogeriatrics: Report of a WHO Scientific Group*. (Geneva: World Health Organization)

World Health Organization (1978). *Mental disorders: glossary and guide to their classification in accordance with the Ninth Revision of the International Classification of Diseases*. (Geneva: World Health Organization)

Yamaguchi, F., Meyer, J.S., Yamamoto, M., Sakai, F. and Shaw, T. (1980). Non-invasive regional cerebral blood flow measurements in dementia. *Arch. Neurol.*, **37**, 410-418

Yates, C.M., Allinson, Y., Simpson, J., Maloney, A.J.F. and Gordon, A. (1979). Dopamine in Alzheimer's disease and senile dementia. *Lancet*, **2**, 851-852

Index

Name Index